JUDITH VON HALLE, ι ̶ ̶̶̶̶ ̶̶ ̶̶̶ ̶ 1972, attended school in Germany and the USA and subsequently studied architecture. She first encountered anthroposophy in 1997, and began working as a member of staff at Rudolf Steiner House in Berlin, where she also lectured. In addition she had her own architectural practice. In 2004 she received the stigmata, which transformed her life. Her first book was published in German in 2005, and she now works principally as a lecturer and author. She and her husband live in Berlin.

By the same author:

THE CORONAVIRUS PANDEMIC

Anthroposophical Perspectives

Two Letters in answer to questions
from members of the Lazarus-John Branch
of the Free Association for Anthroposophy

Judith von Halle

Translated by Frank Thomas Smith

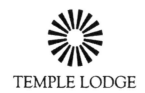

TEMPLE LODGE

Temple Lodge Publishing Ltd.
Hillside House, The Square
Forest Row, RH18 5ES

www.templelodge.com

Published in Great Britain by Temple Lodge Publishing in 2020

Originally published in German in 2020 under the title
Die Coronavirus-Pandemie, Anthroposophische Gesichtspunkte by
Verlag für Anthroposophie, Dornach, Switzerland

A CIP catalogue record for this book is available from the British
Library

ISBN 978 1 912230 54 9

Cover by Morgan Creative
Typeset by DP Photosetting, Neath, West Glamorgan
Printed and bound by 4edge Limited, UK

Contents

II.
QUESTIONS AND ANSWERS RELATING TO ESOTERIC SUPPORT FOR WORK IN THE BRANCH

III.
THE GREAT DIVERSIONARY MANOEUVRE 85

Preface

A great number of scientists, practicing physicians and politicians have spoken about the coronavirus pandemic, which has affected us all and has already made a great impact on our way of life. It is quite a challenge to deal with this flood of information – of course also fortunately made available – to maintain a psychologically healthy attitude. As humanity has come into contact with this virus for the first time, many questions remain unanswered such as its origin and transmission, the prevention of infection or immunity, as well as the treatment of the disease COVID-19, which is caused by the virus. Understandably, this leads to much uncertainty.

One of the strengths of human beings is to face new challenges and to strive for understanding of the unknown with utmost zeal. The search for truth, the dedication to a true understanding, but also to master the circumstances in which we live, drives us forward – especially in this era when the sciences have acquired a dominant position in global society as never before in human history. The endeavour to really understand the coronavirus pandemic or the virus itself is therefore directed mainly towards the sensory-earthly aspects relating to the field of modern science.

That the answers from the purely natural-scientific sector do not satisfy everybody is a gratifying sign that many people are gradually becoming aware that the human being cannot be grasped either in its entirety or in its differentiation by purely scientific criteria. The human soul's natural instinct to understand things beyond the purely scientific fields of research has resulted in countless other personalities appearing on the scene who also wish to help clarify questions relating to the coronavirus pandemic.

Whereas in the field of natural science today – especially medicine and biochemistry – one deals with 'tangible', namely purely material investigative objectives and factors, and exercises substantial expertise in doing so, research in the non-material field almost completely lacks this substantial expertise. The knowledge that the area of the super-sensory can and must be researched using strict scientific methods is hardly present in humanity. And where it is known, what is lacking is the knowledge gained during decades, which as a rule can only be developed over a succession of earthly lives, because the acquisition of super-sensory abilities requires the development over time of the individual I, whereas in scientific work it is sufficient to acquire certain basic knowledge over several years and for everything else to fall back on the achievements of previous generations of researchers.

In my perception, in the current situation of the coronavirus pandemic, this fact represents a further and indeed significant factor of uncertainty and disorientation. For striving to find answers beyond pure natural science often combines unfavourably with inadequate spiritual-scientific expertise, and the need of many insecure souls for quick answers, reasonable explanations and also 'good news'.

To ignore or deny the 'evil' (as it is called in the Lord's Prayer) that is absolutely present and effective in the world is a kind of unconscious reflex action of the soul, when its predominant spirit possesses insufficient knowledge about the relationship of higher and lower moral forces in world affairs. The same cause underlies the apparent opposite, namely the soul's flight to speculative explanations, also known as 'conspiracy theories'. Thus, what is irrational and unprovable mixes with a purely personal way of thinking. The resultant *borscht* may taste good to those who are frightened and hungry for explanations, or to the souls repelled by contemporary science's materialism, but can contribute little or nothing to an objective, spiritual way of considering the problem. Any reasonable person can see that in the field of spiritual-scientific research the human mind is a limited instrument, because of itself it is unable to recognize the mentioned moral – or rather immoral – forces in world affairs, and is therefore the author of personal ideas and convictions that are discoloured by these very forces. But it is just in the present situation – when the willingness to accept this sober (or sobering) insight seems slight – that ever more personalities are able to overwhelm their fellow human beings with unsolicited comments and explanations about the coronavirus question. Curiously enough, it is often the same people who vehemently criticize the media who, without realizing it, use the same methods to enlighten the world about 'the truth'.

Certainly, among the (non-scientific) contributions on the coronavirus pandemic there are also less questionable or even notably constructive considerations, but to my perception these are few because – as mentioned – the obstacles to be overcome in order to present a serious analysis of this question are quite high.

Since I consider my own possibilities in this respect to be quite limited, I originally had no intention of commenting on the coronavirus question and thus presenting yet another version of it to the world. But during the past weeks many people who have read my books or are members of the Free Association for Anthroposophy have come to me with all kinds of questions and urgent requests for my thoughts on the situation. Finally, I could not completely evade these requests and I consoled myself with the thought that it is the task of an anthroposophist not to shy away from the investigation of unknown phenomena, but to objectively investigate them to the point where the individual is in a position to really research them objectively, without making a detour and lapsing into speculation.

However, I wrote my presentation with the intention of using it internally as a kind of interactive contribution exclusively for the members and participants of the Lazarus-John branch of the Free Association for Anthroposophy in the form of a two-part letter – the first part to deal with the questions the participants asked me, as well as aspects of a spiritual consideration of the phenomenon, which I thought to be of interest, whilst the second part was meant to be suggestions for spiritual accompaniment of Branch work during the time of the coronavirus problem. Quite a few of the questions were not only about the difficulty of concentrating on esoteric work in this situation, but also emphasized the question of the consequences of 'social distancing', as well as about the best possible approach to the current restrictions on social life; for the preventive measures decreed by the state, that are meant to hinder the exponential increase of the infection rate in order that care for the sick can be guaranteed, constitute a hard trial for social life. But since social life and its relationships constitute the Christian element of the future, it is clear that the corona pandemic is an attack on exactly this element.

We are certainly far from a Christ-oriented social structure. But perhaps the current restrictions can lead indirectly to the insight that we are far from such a structure, and that social life may have to be built on completely different pillars than on physical contacts alone. Often it is just in the most unfavourable circumstances that the soil is fertile for higher development. To apprehend and use effectively the advantages and chances which come to meet us – whether they are spiritual, psychical (of the soul) or physical – is the task of every individual and of the whole human community. And if they are recognized and accepted, the most difficult trials in life can result in faster spiritual development than would have been the case without them. Seen this way, the human being is never completely subject to outer circumstances.

You will now find that these two letters in the present publication,* in accordance with the wishes of

---

*A third contribution, written as an article and added only to later editions of the original German as an appendix, appears here in Part III.

my [Swiss] publisher Joseph Morel, are available to all who may be interested, instead of only to those involved in its creation. Not only the content itself, but also the form and tone of the personal address of the original letters have been retained. The reason for this is apparent if one considers that the letters offer a means of communication in a completely abnormal situation – for a community which normally meets physically for spiritual interchange.

In ending this preface, I would like to draw attention to the fact that this work, not originally initiated by me, is the result of working with people who are concerned with existential questions related to the current situation. And as is the case with a conversation, the answers given do not constitute a final scientific treatise. That was not the intention. Furthermore, I had important prior commitments, and because the letters had to be sent to coincide with the date of the branch meeting, only three days were available to write this contribution. Obviously a methodical, spiritual-scientific investigation into the coronavirus phenomenon cannot be accomplished in such a short time. Therefore, these observations amount to aphorisms. It is for this reason that this short book is not part of the series of books I have written in the past as mature reflections on certain themes.

Judith von Halle
Berlin, 25 March 2020

I.
WHAT CAN ANTHROPOSOPHICAL SPIRITUAL SCIENCE CONTRIBUTE TO SARS-COV-2 AND COVID-19 RESEARCH?

The First Letter, Berlin, 22 March 2020

Dear Friends!

This rather lengthy letter contains my comments, which you have frequently requested, about the coronavirus crisis. Despite its scope, only a few chosen observations or pieces of knowledge will be indicated. For the time being, all that remains is to open numerous doors without actually entering and inspecting the rooms behind them. But perhaps you will do that.

In that sense, this letter cannot be a final explanation of the coronavirus phenomenon, but rather an interchange with you, thanks to your messages and questions. I am unable to explain the coronavirus phenomenon in all its dimensions. And for this reason I mostly wish to refrain from expressing my personal opinion. In any case, for an anthroposophist it is a purely spiritual-scientific task. To make judgments and give recommendations, especially in the case of important events or situations, demands a scientific background that is supported by a spiritual reality. To investigate the phenomenon in question is a great spiritual challenge which – like the discovery of an effective, classical vaccine – certainly cannot be accomplished in a few days.

Therefore, please accept the following only as motivating fragments for free consideration.

You can also well imagine that during the past days many articles and other contributions, above all by authors from the anthroposophical movement, have been forwarded to me, partly for 'neutral' motives – for my information, and partly from the conviction that the message contains indispensable information about the cause of the illness, evaluation of means to combat it, and so on.

Thereby one can have the impression that – along with several other unfavourable developments – a bad habit has spread which would have been unthinkable in, for example, Goethe's time: skipping over the purely perceptual, unprejudiced observation of a phenomenon and instead judging it immediately, and based on this hasty judgment, acting.

Mixing the process of observation with personal opinions, even if they are based on experience, falsifies the perception. But an unfalsified perception is necessary. For one thing is clear: everything in the world that happens over time is new. There is never a situation that repeats itself exactly; not even in the material natural world (take snowflakes for example) – especially when man as a free responsible being is involved.

To not ignore what is new, with the excuse that nothing different than before will happen, seems to me to be our task in a higher sense as responsible people.

I consider the theories and thoughtless 'actionism' of alarmists and panic-stokers to be just as dubious as those of false saviours and simpletons. Both camps exhibit an undeserved dominance of interpretation and are too quick to tell others 'the truth' without being asked. One is told the *truth*, which mostly means certain people's purely personal opinion.

I consider it even more dubious in this situation – in which what is *new* has not yet been sufficiently phenomenologically observed and researched – when dubious attempts at missionizing are transformed into direct 'actionism'. Even in my own family, we are directly invited to participate in chain letters, signing actions and online petitions, under the motto 'civil liberties' or similar. I find all that seriously encroaching and can recognize little 'liberty' in it.

A look at human history reveals at least one undeniable fact: it has never been proven as constructive to judge or act upon a phenomenon before one has rigorously observed and known its true nature. It seems to me that in respect to the coronavirus neither one has yet happened.

To strive for this knowledge without immediately forming a judgment or an opinion and announcing it to the world should be self-evident to an anthroposophical spiritual student. I mention this to explain why I will not dwell directly or in detail on the many messages explaining the coronavirus and the corona crisis.

As an exception I would like to mention the circular about the corona pandemic from the leadership of the Medical Section at the Goetheanum with the title 'Corona Pandemic – Aspects and Perspectives'

(19 March 2020).[1] It is the official position of the Anthroposophical Society and the responsible Section of the School of Spiritual Science at the Goetheanum for this historic event.

'Corona-Pandemic – Aspects and Perspectives'

About the 'Aspects'

The dominant theme in the circular is the *disposition* of a person for the development of a COVID-19 illness.

Of course the individual disposition for an illness is in no way to be denied. Nevertheless, I consider the emphasis on this aspect in the present case to be questionable for several reasons.

Firstly, because of the emphasis on individual disposition for a COVID-19 illness, the impression can easily arise that the person who develops the illness or who suffers most from it is personally responsible, either because of their comportment in this present life or because of their individual karma; in other words, their condition is due to their 'guilt-account'. In the circular, stress, tension, insufficient sleep and movement, among other things, are named as leading to a higher risk of infection.

By implication one could mistakenly think: whoever doesn't get sick or whoever survives had either behaved correctly in respect to their physical constitution, or in a previous life had acquired a spiritually positive disposition in order to not become ill from the coronavirus in this life, and was therefore a good person in the previous life. In the Medical Section's circular it is not expressed in this way. But one could draw such conclusions from it.

In my opinion a completely different view about karma must be taken here and thereby also about the realm of the Hierarchies.

There is the *individual karma*, the *karma of a people*, and the *karma of humanity*. In the case of COVID-19 all three are undeniably involved, so that the individual disposition is not alone responsible for the eruption of an illness. That 'not every person [...] after an infection [with a virus] develops signs of illness, and if so, then in very differing degrees' is undisputed. But a view to the present situation clearly shows that both the karma of a people and the karma of humanity play an important role.

The assertion is made that it is known that 'with COVID-19 there is a distinctly greater risk for old people and patients with previously existing illnesses...' (apparently for the gravely ill or the dying is meant), based on statistics from China. Meanwhile it has been shown, however, that this does not seem to be the case in such a decisive way for Europeans and Americans. (Munich hospital doctors speak of an even age-demographic distribution of their patients.) So the relationship within Europe might vary, even from country to country. The cause of this can only be determined by spiritual-scientific research.

It is a fact, though, that this is a pandemic event and this means that the karma of humanity is applicable, and it can have happened in such a way that planned individual karma is thwarted. We must realize that after the death of an affected person whose individual karmic threads are severed by the karma of humanity, it is not easy for the Hierarchies to weave these threads back together again.

Of course, each destiny must be considered individually! Nevertheless, the karma of humanity can thwart individual karma to the extent that in individual cases one can come to the conclusion that this person had no individual disposition for the development of a grave illness or for suffering death by COVID-19. If it comes to suffering a misfortune to adjust humanity's karma, other criteria could be used, and if one thinks that because of an unhealthy lifestyle or because of personal karma a person simply had a disposition for dying from COVID-19, it would be the same as the conviction that someone had a disposition to die from a natural catastrophe, as did thousands of others who were not karmically connected to that person.

Precisely in a pandemic, but especially in the case of COVID-19, the disposition is no longer so clearly individualized. Because of this we recognize the signature of the power active here, for it is a full-frontal attack on the I-hood of the individual when karma is thwarted or is downright cut off.

Let us remember that it is mainly the luciferic spirits that act against the astral body, the ahrimanic spirits against the etheric body, and the asuric spirits against the physical body. And against the I? Against the I and the I-Bringer, Christ, acts the being known for that very reason as the Anti-Christ, or also as *Sorat*.

Even if this pandemic causes fewer deaths than other pandemics, as some people claim (albeit without waiting for the provisional end of the pandemic), for purely spiritual reasons it is still a very serious phenomenon, and one differing from most previous illness-causing epidemics. For its attack is by the mightiest spiritual enemy which humanity must face on its path to development. (Even if the SARS-CoV-2 virus is only a rippling wave compared to what humanity must still undergo in the near future.)

It is not only the individual due to his personal biography, but also *humanity as such* that has developed a disposition for illness by this virus in that it has promoted and cherished materialism in its thinking for the past 150 years. One can say that the coronavirus belongs to today's humanity, although that does not mean that it should.

The intensification of this general disposition of humanity's karma is a consequence of the most powerful spiritual nemesis and those submissive beings who serve him, and it will show to what extent humanity – including anthroposophists – is capable of resisting this entity.[2]

A second aspect, from the Medical Section's circular, is that of fear, i.e. that fear of the virus induces a disposition for illness caused by COVID-19. This statement is also correct. Rudolf Steiner indicated that angst and fear of germs during sleep increases one's susceptibility to them. However, is fear of the coronavirus responsible for its exponential, pandemic spreading?

The young people who were on a skiing vacation in Ischgl and are now connected to respirators, for example, obviously had no fear of coronarvirus, for it had appeared in Ischgl a week before the pistes, bars and guest houses were closed. Rather than angst and fear, the problem here appears to be exaggerated carelessness and ignorance concerning the spiritual context as well as the dangers fomented by the adversary powers. The carefree and thoughtless life of a materially-sensuous, so-called fun-loving society on the pistes and après-ski obviously prevailed over fear of the illness. (By the way, I could also say this for a substantial part of the Berlin populace which, according to my observations, move through supermarkets and plazas, weekend markets, streets, parks and woods without the prescribed 'social distancing' or face masks.)

And the elderly, whose immune systems are basically weaker than those of the young, and for which reason they are included in the so-called high-risk group and are known to suffer more often from serious diseases, are conspicuous for showing a certain serenity as well as being less inclined to fear, for in the course of their long lives they have overcome much.

Incidentally, with reference to the elderly we could consider the question of the effectiveness of the body's inflammatory reaction to the enemy invader, which is mentioned in the Medical Section's circular. That anti-inflammatory and anti-pyretic means are counter-productive for an immunological reaction cannot be discounted. However, it is precisely the elderly – who are said to be the most severely affected by the illness – who hardly develop fevers any more. And for many other people too, their physical bodies no longer react in the same way they did twenty years previously. Either they don't react at all to an inflammation or they over-react, that is, the reaction is so strong that a life-threatening condition ensues. A high fever lasting over seven days appears to be an indication of a severe or even fatal progression of the illness. A criterion for an unfortunate result appears to be over seven days of persistent high fever. This is obviously a specific characteristic of COVID-19. But added to this is the fact that today mankind is trapped within a degenerate development, because it does not accept and nurture spiritual life with sufficient dedication. And this degenerate development advances with rapid speed.

In respect to the immune system and the administration of anti-inflammatory medication, more thorough research and differentiation are also required. Whereas it is basically a disadvantage to suppress the immunological reaction by anti-inflammatory medication, an excessive reaction of the so-called immune-system during the later stage of a severe development of COVID-19 is clearly characteristic and presents the attending physicians with a serious problem which they seldom face in cases of classic pneumonia caused by bacteria. In reality it could happen that such reactions of the immune-system – especially in previously healthy young people without pre-existing conditions – lead doctors to give their patients immunity-suppressing drugs in order to gain control of inflammations caused by an extreme reaction of the immune-system, to avoid that becoming the actual cause of death. This is of course like trying to put out a fire with gasoline. For just like a *weak* immune-system, an *extreme reaction* of the immune-system is not one of the essential components of an organism. What is then really meant by the spiritually questionable term 'immune-*system*'? It is a specific activity of the I in the blood. It is not a spiritually uncoupled, purely biochemical *system*, but a highly complex event, enacted by the highest component of the human being. The balancing activity of the I in its physical bearer, the blood, in relation to the invading illness's causative agent, has been undermined for decades – spiritually, psychically and by physical measures such as exaggerated hygiene and the excessive use of antibiotics, so that the I in the blood – the immune-system – has too little to do, so to speak. It is no longer able to recognize what is manifested as good or evil in the world and react in an appropriate way. This results in over-reactions of the immune defenses. The increase in autoimmune illnesses is also related to this. According to my spiritual perception, this is not exclusively a problem of individual disposition, but is also caused by the karma of humanity.

The argument about fear is also, if anything, too weak when considering the outbreak and spreading of the coronavirus in its early phases. It is fully justi-fied, however, in respect to the social and economic effects that result from the restrictions on public life in general.

Although it is also correct to say that fear of eco-nomic loss is detrimental to health, as stated in the circular, fear of economic or social loss due to the prescribed behavioural restrictions meant to contain the coronavirus did not lead to the initial spread of the coronavirus. It was present before the social and economic restrictions.

The fear and feeling of being overwhelmed associated with the projected scenarios, such as the so-called 'worst case scenario', do play an important role for the present and future psycho-physical constitution of humanity.

However, to concentrate on the analysis of fear and feelings of being overwhelmed in respect to the coronavirus phenomenon doesn't seem sufficient. There is also danger in stating that one should have no fear, which could lead to the misunderstanding that the virus in not dangerous (which it is, because, as stated, humanity as such has acquired a disposition for the illness).

Furthermore, due to the unfounded conclusion based on a single statement by Rudolf Steiner that one should have no fear, the impression is created that somehow, someday, everything will be fine. But this would be a fatal error. For nothing will be fine. Human beings must make it fine themselves! Otherwise the consequences for humanity's karma will one day be so far-reaching that incarnations will hardly be possible. That is what will happen if we simply decide that *everything* will *somehow, someday*, be fine again.

Aside from that, it would be foolish not to fear Sorat's intentions. A healthy portion of – not oppressive – fear can be lifesaving. By this is not meant physical life but spiritual life.

So when one says that fear of coronavirus increases disposition for the illness, consequently it means that when one has no fear, it lessens. Naturally this must mean that fear should be replaced by psychical development, through living with spiritual reality, and that this is so essential that thoughts of illness and death don't make one cringe to one's core; rather, that death, however it may occur, is an event which is not so very different from going to sleep at night. (The differences between sleep and death become clear through the inner development that leads to spiritual knowledge in the bright light of consciousness.) Thus, when the immortality of one's own spiritual being is so self-evident that one no longer has to be told, 'Those who believe in me, *even though they die*, will live' (John: 11, 25), then the individual human being can be in total peace when they become seriously ill or physically die, regardless of the cause. Such an inner psychical development can also lead to physical stability, that is, to a lesser disposition to illness.

Fear can therefore only be overcome correctly (in the sense that it also induces real immunological effectiveness), in that one puts something in its place which also has the force to resist the attack to which one is exposed.

Whoever wishes to defend themselves against a soratic infiltration must achieve much knowledge. Furthermore, the basis for a realistic evaluation of the situation – and what can effectively be done against it – requires great respect for the will-impulses of the opposing spiritual powers. Therefore, one must first of all have good reason not to need fear. The person must really have no reason to fear this attack. An auto-suggestive prayer to the effect that one need have no fear will not solve this, nor will it solve the coming challenges, which will derive from the aforementioned spiritual region.

I'll refrain from quoting Rudolf Steiner's relevant statements about bacteria and viruses, which have already appeared in almost all contributions from the anthroposophical scene, as well as in the Medical Section's circular.[3] Nevertheless, although Rudolf Steiner's statement about the 'Lies of Humanity' and their epidemiological importance is cited in the circular, we can wonder why they are not applied to the disposition of humanity as such.

An additional aspect cited in the circular is the reference to 'exposure to the sun' as the basis for strengthening the immune-system. This indication is not gone into more deeply in a spiritual-scientific sense, as it should have been, for otherwise it is a mere general remark with no precise relation to the COVID-19 illness. Apparently, people have long since grasped this connection anyway. Seldom have I seen so many people walking out in the sun since the beginning of the restrictions on leaving one's house.

Perhaps we could conduct a thorough investigation from an anthroposophical viewpoint for the spiritual advantages of exposure to the sun during the corona crisis. The importance of light, the quality of light, knowledge of the quite different entities in light and its intentions and effects and so forth, could be worked out. Otherwise the danger exists that the reference to the beneficial exposure to the sun will be understood only externally. But today human beings *must* learn to *think spiritually* in order to understand *why* light acts beneficially, in order that it can continue to act beneficially from now on. If we do not learn to think about this spiritually, the I remains active only in an unconscious way. And if such knowledge is not achieved and one's view remains confined to the physical plane, at some point the effect of light on the physical organism will no longer be only beneficial. (In fact, this process has already begun.)

About the 'Perspectives'

In the circular under the title 'Perspectives', the physical, psychical and spiritual dimensions are mentioned.

Whereas in respect to the physical it is pointed out that a 'higher consumption of sugar' weakens 'the body's defenses' and the 'absorption of sunlight' strengthens the 'defense against infections', a 'rhythmic daily organization' and 'healthy nutrition' or 'curative eurythmy' are recommended as means of prevention. With respect to the psychical dimension, a 'positive emotional style' is designated as 'beneficial' and leads to less risk of illness, whereby the 'cortisol concentration in saliva' also correlates. Under the aspect of the spiritual dimension, the 'great questions' are presented, a 'growing economic, social and societal threat' is spoken of, as well that the 'relationship of man to the three kingdoms of nature and especially to animals are of great importance' – also the 'necessary new ecological orientation' which could be worked out 'in light of our common cosmic origin'.

At the end it is conceded that the COVID-19 illness 'is still therapeutic uncharted territory for all concerned', but this situation is replied to by: '... in intensive medicine we have knowledge about how to treat respiratory stress syndrome', as well as 'anthroposophical medicine's therapeutic experience in the treatment of ambulatory-acquired pneumonia, which is relatively often provoked by viruses'. Furthermore, 'in our opinion, anthroposophical medicine's therapeutic recommendations can help in all stages of the illness'. (Here the reader might wonder why they don't add, '– at least it probably can't hurt.')

Is that enough? Is this anthroposophical medicine's contribution to the spiritual dimension of the SARS-CoV-2-virus and the COVID-19-pandemic?

When it is said, 'Prevention and healing must therefore also include this spiritual dimension, along with much more', it is likely correct, but it would be more precise – in an anthroposophical sense – to say first that healing is made possible by knowledge of the spiritual dimension of this phenomenon. Because the only effective medicine of the present and future depends on this.

If we don't go deeper into the subject anthroposophically, then the statement that sunlight and a positive outlook are beneficial for health is a mere platitude – no more than a triviality – which is also considered self-evident in hard-nosed, agnostic medical circles.

Allow me here to make a personal remark, which is not meant sarcastically, but derives from a real concern: I don't think this circular will meet with any opposition to speak of from non-anthroposophical conventional medicine, but rather agreement. I do not mean that we have reached a milestone whereby conventional medicine agrees with the statements in the circular and thus recognizes anthroposophical knowledge of man and spiritually-based medical research. Rather, that there are hardly any anthroposophical statements in this circular which contradict medicine based on a purely material *physis*, or nature. For it is specifically about the spiritual dimension of coronavirus that absolutely nothing is said here regarding the efforts of anthroposophical research.

Nobody can justifiably reproach me for criticizing the publications of others in all the years of my work in the anthroposophical movement – the opposite is probably more the case. Perhaps because of this it is clear that what I say here is not personal quibbling, but due to my great concern that Rudolf Steiner's insistence on the spiritual-scientific investigation of new phenomena is insufficiently achieved, if at all.

I repeat that I do not presume to believe that an epochal contribution to anthroposophical research could be achieved in this case, but that one should at least attempt an anthroposophical investigation into this challenge which affects us all.

So much for the Medical Section's circular.

An Attempt at a Deeper Consideration of the Coronavirus Pandemic

If we wish to attempt a deepened consideration many different aspects arise, which I would like to formulate as questions, as you have frequently done in your letters, for example:

- In what way did the virus originate?
- Why does it affect human beings?
- Which human beings does it affect?
- What are the characteristic physiological symptoms–pathogenesis in the body?

The objective outer-sensory and inner-supersensory observation of the phenomenon can begin with such questions. Only then do the moral questions arise. To these moral questions belong the following:

- What are the spiritual causes for the origins of the pandemic?
- How should one behave psychically in this situation?
- Which crises and which opportunities can result from this situation?
- What are the tasks now and for the future?
- Can effective means for treatment and prevention be found that are brought to light by spiritual science?

Answers to the moral questions can mostly be found by supersensory observation of the phenomenon. A subjective-personal moralistic assessment is a hindrance to an unprejudiced perception of the situation. An assessment arrived at in that way is in any case unacceptable. The questions must be answered from out of the higher moral life of spiritual consciousness, for the entire problem in all its facets is a thoroughly moral phenomenon in a higher sense.

What appears in our earthly world as many different aspects but belongs together in the spiritual world, is the essence of a being; and that is how the human soul experiences it when – after death or in meditation – it makes the spiritual world its own. However, here in the earthly world these aspects must be considered first as individual phenomena with specific characters and differentiated from each other; that is, they should be recognized before they can be spiritually assessed together. During this work one must not forget, however, that those aspects never stand for themselves alone, although a structural separation is necessary at first. Otherwise something happens which one must guard against when encountering the spiritual world during the meditative state: everything is mixed up in an impenetrable conglomerate by our own psychical constitution, by our thoughts, feelings and intentions. In this way we do not create an appropriate picture of the object under investigation. In the spiritual reality its various aspects are very well structured and meaningfully merged.

It will not be possible, however, in the short time available for responding to your many messages and questions, to describe this structure. As mentioned previously, this is an aphoristic piece of work that requires your comprehension and adroitness to have value.

About the Spiritual Cause of the SARS-CoV-2-Virus

The greatest difficulty currently facing human beings is that they do not want to acknowledge the I, that is, the reality of their spiritual origin and purpose – the reality of their selves as a community of entities of purely spiritual nature, who at the present time have taken on materially physical sheaths. Only when this insight exists will life on earth for humanity – an existence that can truly be called *life* – be able to continue. For all that we wish to initiate, in research and in practice, requires the clear awareness and understanding that the *invisible* spheres of thinking, feeling and will, as well as the *visible* spheres of nature (mineral, vegetable and animal), stand in an equally direct and inseparable interrelationship.

If one separates these spheres from one another in imagination, today's scientific thinking emerges externally as objective and factual, as incorruptible and free of illusions. Inwardly, the result is isolation from spiritual life – the expressions of which, at a certain point, are driven out and begin to manifest themselves in the physical world as pathogens and illnesses which appear in a living organism and multiply parasitically within it.

A *different* world, which is not included in the divine development plan for humanity, arises through this parasitical isolation. If human beings recognize their I and its importance, its tasks and possibilities, *moral individualization* begins – the self-desired maturity from a creature to a *new* god. If human beings do *not* recognize their I and its importance, its tasks and possibilities, an *amoral special existence* begins, a self-degeneration from divine creature to a *new* – never before existing and also not in a higher sense envisaged – *sub-sensory creature*. Then human beings consummate this splitting from the whole and suck out all they can of the living world that had been bestowed upon them, thus furthering their degeneration.

Objectivity in research, in thinking, is only possible when the person's whole psychical inner world is *not* separated from the physical-sensory objects with which the person is surrounded and interwoven. (For this, good training is of course required, just as good training is needed if one wants to master a craft. For it is important to correctly classify the different connections of the diverse psychical processes and sensory phenomena and to assign them correctly, and not to work with general concepts, as sometimes happens in esoteric circles. A prosaic comparison: If you want to bake a chocolate cake you must use quite specific ingredients. You will not attain your objective if you use sauerkraut and liverwurst and generally claim that baking cakes depends on using foodstuffs.) The synergy of the psychical-spiritual reality with the physical world – one could also say, the sensory-material manifestation of the psychical-spiritual beings and their activities – is so complex that in order to perceive them one must create the corresponding prerequi-sites. But it is precisely this that is the task of the human I since the beginning of the consciousness soul age!

When conducting research into complex events and how to deal with them, people must not only arrive at an initial idea that their inner life and mac-rocosmic life are directly related, but they must also achieve clarity about the details involved by means of spiritual research into the relationship between microcosmos and macrocosmos, and between the (sensory) visible and (sensory) invisible spheres. As far as the coronavirus pandemic phenomenon is concerned, one must by all means try, to the extent one is able, to avoid generalities and to concentrate on truly spiritual-scientific activities.

The cause of this coronavirus pandemic, according to my spiritual perception of the problem, may at first seem to be a cliché, just like one of those gen-eralities. But I can find no other cause. On the con-trary, the cause of few phenomena appearing on earth at the present time are so obvious.

According to my knowledge, the cause is *materi-alism* – which has spread out over the entire earth – and especially in humanity's predominantly *mate-rialistic way of thinking*.

Nevertheless, despite this simple seeming asser-tion, the emergence, progress and effect of the prob-lem is much more complex. And much investigative work is needed to determine the wide ramifiications of this phenomenon. This can be seen by tracing the path that materialism has taken in humanity's development.

First of all, materialism did not just suddenly appear, but different steps for its proliferation – which were taken by different peoples at different times – were necessary. Furthermore, materialism itself was transformed until it has become today's extensive and global worldview. Today theoretical materialism, along with the classic practical version, prevails. In this sense materialism recently passed through a turning point.

The prerequisite for this (although development could have gone otherwise, for man is a free being in the age of consciousness soul development) was the event which Rudolf Steiner called 'the fall of the spirits of darkness' to the earth in the year 1879.[4] At that time the confrontation with the spirits of materialism was definitively set in individual souls, which means that from that point on, every human I incarnating on the earth is confronted with the following question: Along with this sensory world, does a creative spiritual one also exist in which my own being originated, or does it not? Every individual I must answer this question. That this does not happen – with apparently many human 'I's sleeping through this question to the extent that they leave the answer to a few others, namely the fighters for a spiritual worldview, and hence they thoughtlessly and willingly join the materialistic worldview – is cause for grave consequences for human development in respect to the turning point which we have now passed through.

Thus it is materialism in people's perception of the world and of their own actual being which is destructive in a new way.

Without question it is the ahrimanic inspiration – which manifests itself in digital networking and the globalization of information – that has made the spread of intellectual materialism possible in a pandemic way. The material progeny of this intellectual materialism, the coronavirus, has proliferated in lightning quick style and globally.

During the past 150 years, the individual I had the concrete task of cognition, with good conditions prevailing for mastering it. Instead, possessing all the prerequisites for knowing the spirit, it devoted itself to a group ideology, rejecting spiritual reality and the responsibility of the individual for the whole – and thereby a completely new spiritual dimension – and thus assumed the physical consequences. In 1911 Rudolf Steiner drew a simple but clearly understandable diagram on the blackboard (see GA 131, *From Jesus to Christ*[5]):

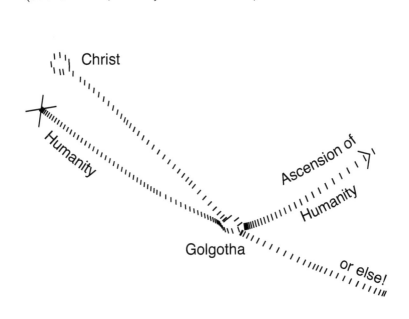

In 1924, in a First Class lesson, Rudolf Steiner named and clearly characterized 'the enemies of knowledge' and their effects (see GA 270, Esoteric Instructions for the First Class of the School of Spiritual Science at the Goetheanum).

We must clearly understand that what is said as the result of spiritual-scientific research is not a mere story or abstract information about which one may philosophize without it having a true meaning for real life – without it being something we feel in our own body. Spiritual science furthers knowledge of the conditions and facts of life on earth, truly felt *within one's own body*. In an age when humanity consists of responsible individuals, the effect of such a rejection of spiritual life is much more serious than at any time in human evolution.

Instead of an I-conducted and free, socially responsible cooperation of individuals, the I-activity has not reached its full potency, so that today there are large associations of people who – well beyond previous epochs when such things were appropriate – maintain a group-soul attitude. In these intelectually-pandemic associations of people, self- and group-needs speak of a corrupted soul activity that has not been conquered by the I.

Up until now, this historical opportunity to awaken awareness and to increase the activity of the consciousness soul in the confrontation with the ahrimanic spirits has not been accomplished. Until this happens many stages must be passed through. Mankind has caused these stages, and they have been promoted by the spirits who wish to paralyze human development.

The kind of materialism we have in the world today is based on a step in development which in itself was not destructive – it was the blossoming of intelligent thinking in ancient Greece during the intellectual soul age. When we speak of such a blossoming, it follows that in the ages that ensued, these blossoms withered and decayed.

What followed is the triumphal march of materialism through European countries, which is responsible for the present virus pandemic. Among other prominent steps on the road to the fading away of the once beneficial intellectual soul culture were the political and cultural seizure of power and Rome's centuries-long dominance of the ancient world; then the takeover of this rule by the representative of the Christian faith, the Roman Church; the powerful spiritual attack on a healthy formation of consciousness soul culture, before the completion of the intellectual soul epoch, by the Academy of Gondishapur in what is now Iran; the second crisis high-point during the time of the persecution of the Templars by the French King Philip IV, through which modern materialism has been developed in relation to which mammon was introduced; and then the strengthening of the Catholic Church in Spain, and Spain's claims to power as well as its unmatched plunder in the New World; the (undisputedly necessary) impulse from Germany and Switzerland for the Reformation, which little by little also took over the Scandinavian countries, the consequence of which meant the total de-spiritualization of the

Christian religion that was a preparation for today's scientific and technological worldview; the perversion of economic thinking in England as well as the incorporation of capitalism in the United States of America; and finally a form of communism manifesting itself in materialism in Russia and in other (now former) communist countries.

These are only fragments of the path which led to today's materialism, and I haven't even mentioned the philosophical-spiritual milestones, but have merely followed a segment of the geopolitical trail. No doubt Europe played the decisive role until this was taken over by the United States of America after the end of the First World War.

When we look for the actual attacks on the consciousness soul impulse, we have not far to look. The allegedly purely objective scientific thinking, and through it the universally-propagated materialistic basic perception of the world and of the human being, determines our everyday world, beginning with school. It has not spared Waldorf schools (exceptions prove the rule), but within a few years Waldorf education in its very essence has been almost completely stifled. Such developments do not take place as if by magic without human involvement; they are brought about by people like us. It can only happen, though, if individuals do not recognize the task that has been assigned to them in their present incarnation. This explains the unthinking adoption of certain judgments and outlooks which cyclically and ever more quickly spread through humanity as comprehensive 'trends'. In a spiritual sense, these are group-soul streams, which are not incorrectly called 'mainstream'. For it is truly a wide stream that carries along all the people who either sleep deeply in their I-consciousness or – if they imagine themselves to be awake – are at least dreaming and therefore do not develop the will to swim against the current.

This mainstream worldview of either an openly declared materialism or of a superficial materialism dressed up with a whiff of rosy esotericism, goes back to seemingly objective scientific thinking, and therewith this materialistic worldview is – like its impulse-giver, the seemingly objective scientific thinking of the present – a bearer of the Gondishapur impulse, which has been revived in this respect. These are enemies of consciousness soul development, which the individual I must seize upon if humanity wishes to one day achieve its earthly goal.

If we look beyond this sketched, fragmentary background to the so-called coronavirus and the pandemic that it has caused – if we recognize the actual cause as the materialistic way of thinking during the present epoch, actually under the impulse of Michael, the true *zeitgeist* of the consciousness soul epoch – then we can, above all if we have understood Rudolf Steiner's corresponding insights, realize *which* spiritual entities inspire current events (and not only these). Since the year 1998 we are in the third cycle of the soratic attack on human development. The first occurred around the year 666 and found its centre in the activities of the

Academy of Gondishapur; the second around the year 1332, when for the first time it expressed itself in people personally steeped in materialism who initiated the obliteration of the Templar Order.

The present third attack by this anti-spiritual power has a different dimension than both previous attacks, because it takes place during the consciousness soul age, a time when the individual potentially possesses the force to oppose that power: one's self or I-consciousness.

This material – but microscopically tiny, diluted to invisibility – infiltration differs from other illness-causing pathogens that afflicted humanity in earlier times. It has – at first only spiritually considered – a different vehemence and meaning, although the threat to human life by viruses is not unknown. For that reason, by overstepping the above-mentioned point in the course of time, and because of the third surge of the Sorat-impulse, it also differs from seasonal influenza epidemics.

In fact, the appearance of so-called human pathogen viruses, that is viruses dangerous to humanity, are a quite recent phenomenon in human history. And, when considering a spiritual-scientific understanding of the present situation, we should concentrate on this point for at least a moment.

In many anthroposophical reflections I have observed so far, there is a tendency to lump bacteria and viruses together due to reference to Rudolf Steiner's formulations. Because bacteria and viruses are – spiritually considered – both of sub-sensory origin, that is, impulses condensed into matter by ahrimanic spirits, this is correct and valid. When considering the present situation more precisely however, it is advisable to differentiate between them.

On the Character of Bacteria

In earlier times and until the recent past, infection pathogens in the form of bacteria (or bacilli) had a different effect on people (above all in spiritual terms). We could even say – broadly speaking – that they fulfilled a beneficial purpose for human development, or at least they could be used by the good divine spirits to dislodge the opposing spirits, in order to arrive at a certain point of development to which humanity had to be brought: namely the point of full earthly self-consciousness. The confrontation with bacteria or bacilli was a kind of (quite unpleasant) offence against the sensory-earthly world, which could be used for the formation of self-consciousness.

During the times when this process was appropriate, an understanding of karma – which today human beings must have in respect to themselves and the world – was not yet applicable. (This is explained in my book from the series 'Approaches to Understanding the Christ Event', Volume 4, *Illness and Healing*, in the chapter entitled 'Illnesses Today' – in contrast to illnesses at 'the turning-point of time'.[6])

Differentiation

The pandemic infections caused by bacteria of earlier ages were a characteristic of the sentient soul age and the intellectual or sensibility soul age. The bridge for their spreading was always the water element, that is, droplet infection or the direct intake of contaminated water.

Let us look for a moment at bacterial plagues in the ages of the sentient soul and the intellectual or sensibility soul, which we can also call illnesses of humanity in its group-soul development phase.

Leprosy
This is relatively less contagious because the only means of transmission is direct contact. These bacteria have played a role as plagues affecting humanity for thousands of years, and they have hardly changed since earliest times. They were dangerous for humanity during the time when the etheric body became more or less congruent with the physical body and the I could insert itself. Around the middle of the fifth Atlantean epoch the conditions were created for these bacteria to become harmful to humanity. The leprosy at that time that is often mentioned in the Bible was a consequence of one's own actions or the actions of relatives within the same lifetime, and was meant as a karmic symbol for understanding in order to prepare the affected person's soul, and humanity, for higher morals. Leprosy's source of contagion is zoonotic (a jump from animal to human).

Plague
This is highly contagious. Close distance is required for contagion through droplets for infection via the lungs. In contrast to influenza viruses, the plague bacteria soon die in the air. Death is caused by an infection of the blood. The original source of the plague is said to be in East Asia in the thirteenth century. An epidemic occurred in the chronological and spiritual aftermath of Sorat's second attack, namely at the end of the fourth cultural epoch.

The cause of transmission is also zoonotic.

Cholera
Here, infection is directly through water contaminated with fecal matter. The most effective treatment is compensating for the loss of liquid caused by diarrhea and vomiting, as well as giving sugar and salts. Although investigators have found evidence of cholera bacteria as far back as 600 BC, the pathogens only became dangerous as epidemics around the turning-point of time. (Again, see in *Illness and Healing* about bathing in the Siloam and Bethesda pools without consequences.)

Typhus
This is one of the infection illnesses that affect the whole organism by a bacillus, a rod-shaped bacterium. It is fecal-oral transmitted, for example by contaminated food or polluted water. It is an inter-cellular pathogen that spreads in lymph and bloodstreams. The so-called Plague of Athens during the Peloponnesian war[7] was clearly a typhoid epidemic. The source of this salmonella pathogen, or

rather the prerequisite for the later epidemic, was the beginning of cattle breeding. Typhus also first became dangerous for humanity around the end of the sentient soul age.

Anthrax
This is an infectious illness caused by the anthrax bacillus, which mostly affects cloven-hoofed animals (even-toed ungulates), but which can also be transmitted to humans. Actually, anthrax should be excluded from consideration, because transmission from person-to-person has not occurred, for which reason there has been no epidemic or pandemic propagation. It is an illness described by ancient Greek and Roman poets.

Tuberculosis
This is induced by mycobacteria, like leprosy. Along with leprosy, perhaps the oldest epidemic of an illness. It is mostly transmitted by droplet-infection. It takes on a new importance in the consciousness soul age, however, namely the first occurrence of the karmic consequences of delusional ideas; since then it is airborne. (Spiritually considered, a certain connection can be seen between bacterial tuberculosis and the viral COVID-19 illness. One could say that the connection consists in a kind of polarity. It is not possible to go more deeply into this aspect here.)

Aside from the fact that bacteria may be called living beings that are capable of cell-building and reproduction through cell division – although the creative forces are not the same as those which act in the procreation of animals and humans! – and have a metabolism, they differ from viruses in their habitus in that the water element plays a significant role in their transmission. And they are distinguished by typical illnesses from before and around the turning-point of time until the beginning of the consciousness soul age, when they had their origin and their 'timely' importance, that is, affecting humanity when it did not yet have the task of I-activity to the extent it has today. The epidemics caused by them – in humanity's group-soul epoch – mostly pertain to the karma of a group or of a people.

Now we can pass on to viruses.

On the Character of Viruses

The virus, as the life-threatening cause of human illnesses *after* the Christ event, is a plague that plays an important role in human development in the consciousness soul age – although not exactly a constructive one. Whereas bacterial infections during the pre-Christian era, and perhaps also up until the advent of the consciousness soul age, could be helpful in the sense that humankind had to become ever more earthly (for humanity had to connect totally with the earthly essence in order to shed it again by means of the spiritual power of consciousness, enriched by I-consciousness, and rise again to the divine heights from which it had fallen), today human beings are no longer served by becoming more earthly. On the contrary, today human beings must become ever more spiritual.

The sub-sensory spirits who wish to dissuade the human being from doing this respond directly to this spiritual epoch of development, acknowledging the failures of the individual human being in relation to his spirit, by the release of particles which are of a much more 'diluted' nature than bacteria. By this is meant not only the physical size of the viruses, which is thousands of times smaller, but also their spiritual and physical structure. As viruses are not made up of cells and have no metabolism of their own, but only a blueprint of their reproduction, which they can actualize within the cell of a so-called 'host', they are not living beings like bacteria (many of which, by the way, play an indispensable role in the human digestion process, which is not the case with viruses). Moreover, viruses maintain themselves by the principle of errors that occur during their copying process and which often result in optimal situations – for them. Thereby they stand in diametric opposition to the basic divine order, namely the principles of truth, beauty and goodness, which are fundamental to humanity's creative power. The cause of cell death in the human body is what optimizes viral existence. This alone directs our attention to the spiritual nature of a virus.

The capacity for reproduction of human cells – the basis for the effectiveness of productive creative forces within the physical body – is misused by the virus for the replication of its own programme, its own nature. Therefore it is not a case of substantiality as such, but rather of a kind of physical carrier of sub-sensory, counter-spiritual impulses (thinking and will impulses) which are infiltrated into the deepest nature of a living organism.

The basis for the emergence of viruses came about during the dawn of the present incarnation of the earth with the entry of the most powerful spirits in the depth of the occult earth-body, which are part of the seven-stage earthly development: the *asuras*. Through their intrusion in a humanity becoming earthly, in the foundation of its material *physis* (DNA and RNA), something of the original divine spirituality, which underlies this material *physis*, was separated in order intentionally to return it to humanity at a later time, namely in the form of the blueprint for viral reproduction. But because of the separation, and the occupation of the separated portion by the spirituality of the asuras, the separated portion is no longer *human*. It is no longer a living part of the human physical organism when it is brought into contact with that organism again. However, because its genetic material is, so to speak, related to that of the human being, it exerts enormous will-power on the human body.

Thus something almost impossible in the ecosystem became possible: there are organic objects which carry within them the plan for their own reproduction, independent of the actual living organism from which they separated. In order to implement this, however, they utilize the parasitical creative force in every living organism over which the asuras do have power of their own accord, because they had not completed their I-development during the ancient Saturn period, so they cannot inject reproduction forces into the viruses. Reproduction in the cells of the host is, spiritually seen, only a vehicle for transporting a spiritual, or rather a sub-spiritual – in a higher sense amoral – impulse into humanity. During its incarnation it must connect its actual spiritual being with the physical-material element, and thus forms physical-material mental concepts about it. An infection with the virus steers the I-slumbering person's attention back to the purely material-physical processes, and it reaffirms his or her already biased materialistic worldview. It impacts a spiritual (sub-sensory-spiritual) impulse on the physical in the human soul.

What the re-infiltration of the components of the physical bodily and reproductive functions – originally derived from the DNA of early human beings – means for humanity cannot be explained here.

However, with regard to the mechanism of action that occurs, it may be possible to think of an autologous blood transfusion, in which one's own blood that was previously taken is returned to the organism at a later point in time – but because of the spiritual separation of the blood and the resulting killing of the spirit contained in it, which continually burdens and weakens the immune system – the organism would consider the donation of blood to be a life-long enemy to be fought against.

A viral infection has no physical benefits for a person, even if they are officially declared *immune* after overcoming the inflammatory reaction that follows the infection. A viral disease always leaves scars and thus limitations in the etheric body – unless the person is so far advanced due to their consciousness soul activities that they are beginning to transform their etheric body into *life-spirit*.[†]

[†] This note is in reply to letters from members to which I was to give my opinion, with the tenor: the coronavirus is a gift from the higher spiritual powers, which we should not reject, but embrace. To clarify: All physical phenomena of the sensory world are manifestations of certain spiritual and therefore moral impulses, that have very different qualities, which human beings of the consciousness soul age are called upon to recognize and to differentiate; and that viruses – including Sars-CoV-2 – belong to those manifestations of spiritual impulses that are opposed to humanity's higher development. That is the basis of this general explanation.

That combating a viral attack on a child at a certain phase of development can help it gain a foothold on earth and thus be better armed against other kinds of opposing forces that will confront the child on its path of development – compare Rudolf Steiner's indications concerning all kinds of children's diseases such as measles, for example – does not change the fact that the moral (or immoral) spiritual nature of viruses is antagonistic to the higher development of humanity As Goethe's Mephistopheles admits: 'I am a part of the force / that always wants evil and always creates the good...'

Taking advantage of a virus infection refers to the 'becoming earthly' of the person and therefore relates mostly to the development of the child (see also page 57). As manifestations of ahrimanic (not luciferic) impulses, they *promote* deeper bonding with the incarnation.

Of course, man wants to go through more incarnations on earth, but since the event of Golgotha, and especially since the beginning of the consciousness soul age, human beings want to gradually loosen their physical existence from the binding power of the material earth. The human being therefore wants to become a spiritualized earthly person, wants (as a first step) to raise his physical corporeality to the etheric level. (See Rudolf Steiner's indications about the so-called phantom of the physical body in his lecture cycle *From Jesus to Christ*, GA 131.) It is just this higher development of the human being's physical body, which follows in parallel the etherization of his physical earthly body, that will be attacked from certain sides, among others by viral pathogens. The 'scarring' or hardening resulting from viral infections are meant by the opponents to make the activity of higher consciousness in the physical body difficult, and in this way results in the spiritualized body, which requires the knowledge and force of will of the I to 'energize', not being formed. Realizing that such a spiritualized bodily form will be the foundation for all future development of the human being allows us to know what these attacks mean.

The spiritual intention of viruses, as spirit bearers (or non-spirit bearers) reduced to a minimum in material terms, is to cause maximum harm in that they come into contact with the spirit of the human being at the level of *devachan* – albeit at its amoral mirror-image plane – but with the spirit not used by that person. Thus they are a plague of the consciousness soul age.

Virus epidemics affect the *karma of humanity* insofar as the individual spirit is not brought to bear within an individual human being, and as a result, in what is meant to be the age of spiritual awakening, the person relapses into group-soul attitudes, which increase the physical potency of viruses.

A consequence of successful, individual spiritual awakening would have been the Christ-oriented association of 'I's in the sense of the threefolding of the social organism. Instead, because of individual 'I's being asleep, humanity continues to be committed to the group-soul impulse. It had once already suffered from a group-soul karma, namely with the *Spanish flu*, which began to spread towards the end of the fateful year of 1917, and which laid the foundation-stone for the current *soratic* attack in human history.

Due to time limitations, smallpox epidemics cannot be discussed here. Only one aspect, which comes into consideration in respect to combating the coronavirus, should be mentioned as it belongs to the history of smallpox. At the end of the eighteenth

---

Because these attacks have taken on a new dimension since the impact of the third soratic impulse, that is, since the second half of the twentieth century, the effect of the viruses appearing today is also different, as has been described in previous chapters.

century, vaccination against the spread of the small-pox plague was initiated. After the great smallpox epidemics that spread through humanity between the sixteenth and eighteenth centuries came to an end with the vaccination law of 1874, the smallpox virus nonetheless split into two strains. This raised questions about the consequences of vaccination as protection. That vaccination cannot offer lasting protection is indicated by the impulse to mutate that was induced by vaccination. Spiritually considered, vaccination campaigns, however beneficial they may be at first, cannot remedy humanity's karmic adjustment caused by a viral epidemic. At best, a postponement of humanity's karmic adjustment takes place. If the spiritual causes of the plague are not remedied but instead comprehensive vaccinations are administered, a more drastic consequence or compensation must be reckoned with in future.

This is not an appeal against vaccinations. It is only meant to indicate that vaccination campaigns alone are not a solution, but at most a stop-gap, because without the removal of the spiritual causes for the infectious illnesses, they contribute to the eruption of other more powerful epidemics.

The Way SARS-CoV-2 Spreads

The spiritual problem, that is the degeneration of human thinking in the sense of the ahrimanic-coloured worldview, is now characteristic of the new coronavirus – which is asserting itself for the first time since the third soratic attack – with the possibility of transmission from droplet to the *airborne* method. It uses the *air-element* as a bridge from person to person. It is thereby much more contagious than previously recognized or officially declared.

The physical manifestation of the general sphere of thought is the air-element. The physical manifestation of the general sphere of feeling is the water element. The physical manifestation of the sphere of will is the warmth element. Beginning with the thinking sphere, these spheres must, by the individual's activity (through conscious I-activity), become so individualized that they receive a new constitution, which corresponds to the ascending parabolic branch of human development, which no longer follows the Alpha path to the densification of creation, but to the Omega of spiritualization.

Just as we need uncontaminated air to breathe, we need uncontaminated thinking in order to live.

Today we experience the attack – caused by us, as the organism of humanity – on the air-element and the physical organ associated with it, the lungs, through our corrupted, not-life-giving thinking. But if in the future, in the age of the consciousness soul, humanity has sunken so low that it is just as degenerate in its feeling as in its thinking, an attack on the heart will follow. Then it will be a case of lacking compassion, which is connected, among other things, with the suffering of animals.

On the Symptoms of the COVID-19 Illness

Conspicuous among the COVID-19 symptoms are large, extensive – and therefore different from classic pneumonia – milky appearing areas in the *lungs*.

The lungs become rigid (no longer elastic), a disturbance occurs in the pulmonary alveoli's transfer of oxygen to blood circulation, which has a sclerotic characteristic in the case of COVID-19. A point can be reached when even a maximum amount of oxygen does not help because it never gets into the blood. For this reason the ECMO procedure (Extracorporeal Membrane Oxygenation) is sometimes used, by which blood is mechanically enriched with oxygen *outside* the body, or a gas substitute is used as the patient's own respiratory system can no longer achieve this.

What is going on here? First of all, the fixed ideas of materialism eventually put the lungs in this sclerotic situation. Furthermore, today's kind of materialism leads to obsessive thoughts that force people to become addicted to the materialistic worldview. The I is undermined, compelled by its rigid, fearful intellectual soul that has been abandoned by its higher spirit through materialism.

A life of *free* thinking is no longer possible – just as the lungs, when they become stiff and no longer pass oxygen on to the blood, can no longer dynamically relate to the outer world. The human being basically breathes in his own fixed ideas, which causes his breathing organ to become rigid. If the thought-ether is no longer permeated by reality, the air breathed by us will consist exclusively of mere chemical gas. Instead of being the bearer of super-sensory living forces, it will become the bearer of sub-sensory impulses in the form of damaging material particles. The physical breath of life, previously the guarantor of human life on earth, would in this way become a potential menace to life. The cause is I-benumbed thinking, the opposite of what happens when the human being uses what Rudolf Steiner characterized as the (selfless) I-sense.

When we breathe in, we inhale what others have exhaled. In the breathing process we are therefore natural social beings. But when materialistic thoughts are thought again and again, until they have developed dominance over non-materialistic thoughts and develop a kind of independent existence, then this process goes a step further. What does it mean, then, if the perverted, I-coercive intellectual soul activity reduces or blocks the lungs' functioning? It means that what at first took place in the astral body and was limited to the astral body (in a previous incarnation), now appears a stage deeper – pushed down to the next stage. The materialistic concepts about man and the world that were enthusiastically absorbed during the nineteenth and twentieth centuries, have today already sunk into the etheric body.

The following phenomenon, which had not yet appeared in human development until several decades ago, can be considered. Due to the ahrimanic acceleration of all earthly-sensory processes – which, with a powerful impulse of will, forces the earthly-sensory elements and thereby the world's development ever more quickly into rigid degeneration (compare this with the so-called *freezing* in Parkinson syndrome, which ultimately is nothing more than the quickening of a tremor till rigidity) – the time between incarnations has dramatically shortened.

The current youthful generation is in part already in its third incarnation since the spiritual event of 1879! This has been enabled in an untimely way by the termination of millions of lives during both World Wars. But this means that the people who now live on earth (all generations) have already absorbed intellectual materialism in their astral bodies in a previous incarnation. And now, with a damaged organism, in which the pictorial-imaginative mode of thinking is already manifest in the etheric body, they have come to earth again. What was still an intellectual illness, an infection of the intellect in a previous incarnation, in the present incarnation creates the conditions for the destructive effect of that self-enabled intellectual materialism in the physical world: the sub-sensory homunculus, the virus. It is actually the same people, the same individuals incarnated today, who are confronted with their own ideas from a previous life within the karma of a group, or the karma of humanity. (Here lies the connection between bacterial tuberculosis and the viral COVID-19 disease.)

That the imaginative, pictorial aspect in the etheric body appears suppressed – and in a pandemic-comprehensive sense – is shown by the sonographic images of the lungs of the gravely ill. But not only of the gravely ill; also of people who do not notice a serious impairment of their lung activity. This is a milk-like opacity of the tissue, like a fibrosis, which seems to be responsible for the rigidity, the sclerotic tendency of the lungs. It is a phenomenological and true picture of pandemically-pervasive intellectual materialism. The contemporary etheric body has been damaged by the pathological activity of the astral body in one's previous incarnation and is now receptive for what manifests itself physically today as virus – i.e. to what was introduced into the general sphere of thought by one's own astral body in one's previous incarnation.

Spiritual Aspects

Today, we must learn to understand the relationship between macrocosm and microcosm, whereby by macrocosm the earth organism is meant and by microcosm the human being. The psychical-spiritual human being, but also the physical one, has a direct relation to the occult interior of the planet. If consciousness penetrates into the secrets of the sixth occult stratum, it enters the domain of earth-remembrance, which relates chiefly to the cosmic epoch of Old Sun. In contrast to Old Saturn, on Old Sun the unity of the whole – which on Old Saturn was spoken of spiritually as what we today perceive on earth as the warmth-element – divided into two *essential substances*: air and fire. From the earthly standpoint, where we know the four elements as separate states, we can, as Rudolf Steiner did, designate these *essential substances* of Old Sun as *water-air* and *fire-earth*,‡ because at that time air contained what would in future be water and fire contained what would in future be earth-solidity.

---

‡ *Wasserluft und Feuererde.*

The essential substance of water-air – which with the appearance of the fourth earthly incarnation, the present Earth, was repeated in degraded form as *Ruach*[§] – connected with the gradually developing human being on earth. It became, so to speak, flesh, in the *sense of smell*, which first developed on the present earth.

The sixth stratum, the fire-earth – which within today's earth represents the ahrimanic spirits' domain and through which disturbances are generated on the earth's surface by materialistically thinking and willing people – does not only cause volcanic activity and earthquakes. It also affects the microcosm, humanity itself. Humanity responds to the fire-earth within the macrocosmic earth, the microcosmic human body, to the part of itself that binds humanity to the water-air being, namely to *Ruach*. This disturbance of the fire-earth resonates in humanity's *sense of smell*.

In this way both inherited traits of Old Sun, fire-earth and water-air are brought back together, but in a destructive way. One can see in this an indication of the spiritual reason why many COVID-19 patients temporarily lose their *sense of smell*. Whereas *Ruach* (the water-air being not yet permeated by human consciousness) brings the intellectual soul activity to the human soul during the earthly incarnation, the *functioning* activity of the sense of smell is by contrast an activity of the human consciousness soul.

[§] 'The water-air being not yet permeated by human consciousness' – see next page.

If we wish to initiate a healing process, we should strive to advance in psychical-spiritual training to the point where our consciousness reaches the *seventh* earthly stratum, the *earth-mirror*. For there we gain entrance to the forces of Old Saturn, in which water-air and fire-earth (light and air or fire and air) were once united, in an all-embracing state of psychical warmth. (In my view there are indications here for anthroposophical medicinal research.)

If one reaches this psychical-spiritual stage of consciousness, one connects with the *Archai*. It was they who, during the period of Old Saturn, planted the seeds for the human being's future sensory organs.

But the Archai are also the patrons of anthroposophy, so to speak. They are the administrators of cosmic intelligence, of the living spiritual thoughts to which individuals can connect within themselves. That is why they were designated the Spirits of Personality. The connection to the prevailing Archai, who stand opposed to the impulses of the asuras, is a sure prevention against viral infectious diseases.

The *sense of taste* has apparently also become limited in some patients. The sense of taste, like the sense of smell, is an *inner-outer sense*, and is therefore based on the exchange between what comes into a human being from the outside world as a volitional expression of a spirituality working in material, and the activity of the astral body, which is sent to meet this spirituality coming from the outside in order to absorb it within itself and obtain information about it. The relation between the inner and outer worlds is shown in the COVID-19 illness as an additional symptom affecting the senses, which actually ignites the consciousness of the ego. In this way the person is cut off from perception of the outer world.

The impairment of both of these senses by the illness also points to the elementary means used by the virus for person-to-person transmission. With respect to the sense of smell, which is the result of inhalation, it is the element of air; with respect to the sense of taste, which would not be able to function without salivation, it is the watery element, i.e. the transmission of the virus through the so-called droplet infection.

Additionally, it doesn't seem impossible to me that the impairment of the senses of taste and smell has to do with another aspect, which is, however, directly related to this. In my view this phenomenon can be the result of the level of copper in the nervous-sensory apparatus, in the brain. It has not yet been determined whether COVID-19 causes long-term damage, not only to the lungs but also to the brain. But for now, let us return briefly to the copper aspect.

During spiritual contemplation, certain essential helpful effects on the constitution of the present human *physis* and for the organism suffering from COVID-19 were observed; essential effects such as derive from the spiritual domain of the planet Venus. I had to wonder: Why do these seemingly helpful effects from that domain emanate to a such a degree during the present virus pandemic?

In the further pursuit of these essential effects – which at present are particularly directed towards the human being – I came to the following (the spiritual chain of effects going backwards, so to speak, to the causal problems, which are obviously meant to be alleviated by these essential effects):

When the spiritual effects from the domain of the spiritual beings on the earth connected to occult Venus meet, they condense – as do all astral effects – into certain etheric processes within the material cosmos, which in turn correlate with certain physical-sensory – that is, chemical – substances in the mineral basis of the earth as well as in the human biological organism. The original spiritual effects find their sensory expression in these processes and their related substances. Here our attention falls on copper and the enormous role it plays in the human organism.

Copper is particularly dominant in the liver, which is responsible for metabolism. If the human being breathes in his or her own materialistic-egoistic thoughts, as previously indicated, the spiritual development of those forces which work in the liver during the foetal stage is displaced to the lungs. The foetus *must* be materialistic-egoistic, so to speak, because the human being in the foetal stage is composing itself to develop from a purely spiritual being to an earthly one. For this, it must first make everything its own, ingest all the forces and substances for its own use in order to become an autonomous physical-earthly being.

This process is manifested in the growing child in its relatively large liver and its high copper levels. When a person grows up, this spiritual-physical dominance of the liver should recede, for the individual must come into contact with the outer world with the higher members of his being, first through the astral body, then through the I, so that he gradually returns – but now consciously – to being a social and spiritual entity within earthly existence. This is where breathing comes into consideration. The activity of the lungs virtually replaces the dominance of the liver.

If, however, today, through the problems indicated, the one thing takes place spiritually in the human being from which we must free ourselves through growing up – namely through breathing, in which we give out our own being and take up the being of our human brothers and sisters and the world – this will draw our breathing down into the metabolic area – more precisely: metabolic processes shift up into the lungs. What happens is that processes are manifested in the lungs which should remain in the metabolism.

Metabolism takes place in a certain environment, the etheric expression of which are the digestive juices. What is actually apparent in many patients suffering from COVID-19 is the aforementioned flat, milky-white change in the lung tissue. This is a reflection of the milky-white chyle, the digestive juices, and this causes coughing, pneumonia, as well as a disturbance of the thermal balance.

For this reason it seems to me that one could therapeutically treat a COVID-19 patient via the gut – thus 'retroactively' – using a certain kind of copper-therapy where possible. For copper has a tendency to move from the sulphuric toward oxygen, which could be utilized to strengthen the breathing system. There are many other aspects involved however, which I cannot elucidate here, for example the form toward which copper is exposed within the mineral world, namely to the typical bulb-shaped aggregates of malachite. This encapsulated form toward the outer world is, however, constantly overcome by the spiritual force of the Venus-being within earthly copper, as these effects go steadily beyond this spherical, capsule-shaped form. Here, in my opinion, lies an occult connection also to protein synthesis within the liver as well as to the spiky glycoproteins on the covering of SARS-CoV-2 viruses.

I am neither a physician nor a chemist. Therefore my ability to say something more specific and precise – especially within such a narrow time frame – is hardly possible. Appropriately trained and knowledgeable scientists, who are open to such spiritual-scientific considerations, could perhaps elaborate something more concrete in this field.

Among other things to be considered is finding a certain copper-therapy based on homeopathic preparations. If one observes the effect of continuously administering cupric salt to healthy people, namely an uncontrolled activity of the astral body in the nervous-sensory system in which the I cannot intervene, which is reflected, among other things, in the inability to concentrate, to observe one's thinking and to turn to higher viewpoints, and in forgetfulness and angst – then you get to what in the present is the consequence of several incarnations engaged in materialistic thinking.

Commentary on Further Questions

About Animals
On the basis of the results of my efforts to provide a first spiritual-scientific consideration of the coronavirus phenomenon, I cannot see that animals stand in the foreground of the problem. There have always been zoonotic pathogens, even during the early stages of human history. In the future they will take on great importance – but what stands in the foreground of the CoV-2-Virus according to my perception is the karmic consequence of contemporary humanity's mode of thinking. The current viral epidemic is the result of a problem of thought, from the thinking of humanity as a whole in a phase of human development during which this kind of thinking should not be present in such strength and propagation. Hence propagation by the element of air.

In addition, if we consider the smallpox virus as well as the virus that caused the Spanish flu, we are looking at a time when the tortuous breeding practices and massive industrial animal factory farming, to accommodate the so-called affluent society, did not yet exist in this way.

The karmic compensation for the tormenting of animals lies in humanity's future. Completely different problems will then occur, for which materialistic adjustments are already beginning to be made (for example, the development of synthetic foodstuffs). General *feeling* will cause the catastrophe and accordingly the attacks, and the dangers to humanity will be correspondingly much greater than the current (initial) karmic consequences of materialistic thinking.

In my view, in the case of the coronavirus pandemic, what should be considered in respect to humanity's behaviour towards animals is something different than cruelty. What is at issue here, as I said, according to my perception, is a problem of thinking. The human being declares himself to be the highest *animal*. We were taught that already at school. Actually we don't have to be taught it *expressis verbis*, because as a child we are taught it through the behaviour of our parents, which reveals their attitude of thought. If the human being is described as a member of the animal kingdom, as a higher animal, and we let our descendants grow up in that sphere of thought, so the growing human being incorporates within himself what *is* – spiritually considered – of an animal nature. In reality, because humanity left the animal stage behind (as Rudolf Steiner expressed it) in order to become a human being, and since, in contrast to the animal, we therefore have an individual ego, we can therefore fall fatally ill with the coronavirus infection. The animal cannot. In a higher sense this has moral connotations.

Only Hysteria?
Assertions that there are many worse things that happen in the world than the spreading of the coronavirus, or that the coronavirus is nothing

more than a seasonal flu, reveals not only a lack of observational will, but above all a basic lack of spiritual insight. Nobody is served by comparing apples with oranges. On the other hand, if someone comes up with a spiritual-scientific justification for that assertion, I would be glad to question my own spiritual-scientific research results.

The Social and Economic Consequences
Relating to contemporary events, the above were foreseen by the opposing spirits and to that extent also intended. If one does not deny the spiritual reality, one can easily perceive that these spirits hope for a strengthening of materialistic egoism in humanity. The blatant naming of this goal by human mouthpieces ('America first!') shocks no one anymore. Certainly, the social and economic consequences are the counter-image of the framework for social threefolding. The repeated public mentioning of the two areas of social and economic life also reveals the widespread ignorance of spiritual life, which is characteristic of the present attitude and the cause of great misery.

The Question about the Eurythmic Impulse Against the Background of the Coronavirus Pandemic
This is a very legitimate question – casting light on man's maladjustment to his or her bodily and spiritual being. Whereas eurythmy is an artistic and thereby living and enlivening activity of the etheric body, today's mania for sport constitutes an artificial and therefore dead activity of the physical-sensory body, thereby sickening the etheric body. Eurythmists

should take care that they possess a thorough knowledge and understanding of anthroposophy, otherwise eurythmy also threatens to degenerate into a purely physical activity. (This of course does not only apply during the coronavirus pandemic!) Supported by this knowledge and understanding of Rudolf Steiner's anthroposophical research, spiritual research for a curative-eurythmy therapy in the context of the COVID-19 illness could be undertaken, for which, however, a greater understanding by patients of the spiritual roots of such a therapy would be necessary, for – as already stated – the COVID-19 disease is based on the widespread ignorance of spiritual reality.

The Question of Why Children do not Become Ill
I can neither confirm nor give a comprehensive response to this question, but can only say that in the course of my spiritual-scientific efforts concerning the karma of humanity, which indicates materialistic, corrupted thinking, it has been shown that the acquired etheric disposition for an illness through this thinking (that is, from the virus emerging because of it) is present from birth on, so children should also potentially be susceptible to the illness. Perhaps the inclusion of the astral body is needed for a serious illness or death to result. This occurs around fourteen years of age, or somewhat earlier today because of the aforementioned ahrimanic acceleration.

Additional Questions
Further questions I have been asked relate to what could be the object of spiritual work when once

again the time comes that we will be able to meet physically in the branch. This could include on the one hand the overcoming of fear and the disruption of meditative practice due to the current events, as well as the question of the means of obtaining the force for renewal after enforced physical isolation, which also entails the shutdown of cultural, religious and artistic activities in public.

II.
QUESTIONS AND ANSWERS RELATING TO ESOTERIC SUPPORT FOR WORK IN THE BRANCH

Publisher's Note

Part I contains fundamental viewpoints which are answers to questions written by members of the Free Association for Anthroposophy, and are probably also of general interest. The content and form of the following letter is, however, especially addressed to members of this association of people which, as an independent branch within the anthroposophical movement dedicated to the living apprehension and nurturing of the mystery of Christ, meets biweekly. Because this spiritual work is no longer possible during the period when meetings are prohibited, the members directed their questions about the current situation to Judith von Halle.

Joseph Morel
Dornach, 9 April 2020

The Second Letter, Berlin, 22 March 2020

To the Members of the Free Association for Anthroposophy, Dornach

Dear Friends!

Here is the second letter relating to our esoteric work. (The *first* letter, in which at your request I responded to your questions about the corona pandemic, I wrote under pressure of time in two or three days and delivered as promised, but my publisher held it back, because in his opinion it has become a small book instead of a *letter*; he wishes to publish it as soon as possible.) First of all, however, in *this* letter I will address some of your questions about the psychological side of the coronavirus pandemic.

Overcoming Fear

Something was already said about this in the first letter. The real, deeply perceptive embedding of our soul in Christ pours a deep inner freedom into our hearts, which during our life on earth threatens to be dragged down through external hardships and turmoil. But one can say: the worst that can happen to me is that I die from the COVID-19 virus. This may be an unfavourable constellation of fate for the fulfilling of an individual karmic plan, which may have to be corrected or compensated for somehow in one's next life. But it is probably not so much the prospect of this problem that makes us afraid of the virus, but rather the fact that we would have to be very clear about our karmic life plan, and if we had that, we would have reached a stage in our soul's development where such fear is no longer relevant.

So it can only be the prospect of death itself that triggers fear.

But it is just here that the anthroposophical spiritual student has a great advantage. He or she can actively permeate their feelings with spiritual-scientific knowledge about the essence of death and postmortem life. And this says, basically, that death is the most uplifting moment of life, that it is the gate through which we may return to our true homeland, in which we are suffused and redeemed by the inexhaustible love of our divine source – and, moreover, through this permeating love our understanding of the context of cosmic-being grows, so that we feel ourselves to be immersed in a radiant, redeeming light in which the distressing questions of the earthly mind are, so to speak, simultaneously answered – whereby in turn the resulting fears and worries are completely taken away from us. And the thought of being united after death with the loved ones who preceded us can awaken an unbounded anticipation for the moment of crossing the threshold.

For this reason there is nothing to fear – on the contrary. (And – pardon the straightforwardness – the eventual prospect of death by COVID-19 and the preceding suffering should also not particularly burden us, for compared to other ways of suffering before crossing the threshold, as a rule it is limited to several days. Apart from this, the steps we take on our psychical path of inner development awakens with feeling the awareness that our suffering is among the most valuable experiences of this incarnation, for it gives us the opportunity for real insight into the purpose of incarnation.)

When fear grips us, let us look at Christ! Why is it said that He was the first to rise from the dead? Because we ourselves are the second ones to whom this is given. If we contemplate the Easter depiction of the Isenheim altar, it can call upon our souls: See, human being, that is your gift!

How Intensifying Meditation Can be Helpful in These Times

This question will be answered by the following suggestions for spiritual work.

It cannot be dismissed out of hand that the flooding of the soul with information by the media – mostly frightening reports, even when real situations are described – does not only instill anxiety, but also paralyzes activity in that the earthly intellect is constantly occupied with new (or old) information. Here, the only thing that helps is to reduce one's exposure to news about the coronavirus pandemic to the minimum that is necessary to avoid ignorance of what is going on in the world. Rudolf Steiner, alongside his spiritual research, always made sure that he was thoroughly informed about outer events and opinions, because for spiritual-scientific research it is essential to know about outer events, as they constitute the basis for investigation into their spiritual background. After all, spiritual science exists in order to correctly observe and classify the events on the physical plane. However, each person must decide for themselves on the amount of information they require. One needs more, another needs less. This also expresses the responsible, i.e. I-conscious, approach to the challenges of everyday life.

What Does It Mean When People Can No Longer Meet?

This and similar questions which relate to our spiritual work were asked by several members. The human being clearly did not come into the world to keep the most physical distance possible from his or her sisters and brothers! Incarnation itself already separates people from each other however, at least compared to life in the prenatal (or postnatal) spiritual world. We are – at least the karmically connected ones – so closely connected there that one must speak of a permanent permeation (penetration) – although in freedom. This permeation is the most complete apprehension of one's actual being and destiny in relation to the needs of others. This awareness is no longer possible once we descend into material corporeality and become aware of ourselves within it. For that, one must guide one's innermost being, one's ego, out of one's physical dwelling. This is still seldom done, but it is our pre-eminent task in this contemporary epoch of development.

In the limitations on our freedom during this present misfortune, there also lie certain opportunities. We can practice (in the sense of the I) becoming more conscious of the nature of interpersonal permeation. We could say to ourselves, conversely: The dead, the people living in the spiritual world, have no physical bodies. Nevertheless, for this very reason they come into contact with each other (and with us here on the earth) more intensively. Because of the lack of physical meetings, the possibility of coming into contact with each other is in no way lost.

One can think of the explanations in Chapter XIV of Rudolf Steiner's *The Philosophy of Freedom* or of how Jacques Lusseyran dealt with his destiny; how he, as a blind man, was confronted with the cruel, apparent hopelessness of being interned in a concentration camp. He neither died and nor did this destiny break him internally. Not everyone can boast of such inner strength, but achieving it is the goal of anthroposophical spiritual students who draw from their trust in and knowledge of spiritual reality – namely, the everlasting triumph of the immortal spirit over exterior conditions.

We may ask ourselves what do we miss during the curtailment of our physical social contact? If we are honest with ourselves, we would then have to admit that direct social contact is usually utilized to talk a lot. (This is, of course, apart from the undeniable beauty of the sensory, supersensory perception of another's physical nature or by directly perceiving their etheric auras.) In other words, all too often one merely asserts oneself. This must not necessarily be wrong or bad. But when we perform our daily retrospection, we are often painfully moved by the fact that – from the perspective of the spiritual world of truth – we have used only the briefest portion of time available to dedicate ourselves to what is truly meaningful and sustainably beneficial.

Direct physical contact is downright necessary when one is not completely conscious of one's activities and pays a lot of attention to external, superficial things. When we perceive human beings physically, much attention is paid – unconsciously – to their shape, gestures, countenance (through which the soul is naturally also revealed) and to everything else external – that they scratch their head, that they have a new hairstyle or glasses, that they serve tea, etc.

When we eliminate all those things, as right now it's impossible to perceive them, as well as all the superficial and superfluous communications, what's left? To be honest: little. This vacuum in relation to one's own real perception of the other, that is of the other's true nature – to admit this to oneself for once and to recognize in it the necessity to develop the real will impulse to fill this vacuum with spiritual substance – can enable us to counter the intentions of the opposing powers.

Of course, we can wonder how we can perceive the other if we cannot communicate with them in the conventional way. In fact, this is easily possible at a certain stage of inner development without external means, that is with purely psychical-spiritual means! The possibility opens to understand what is essential for the other and what moves him or her. We begin to have a clear life of thought, a true life of thought, and we approach the possibilities that one has after death. In this way it is easier to increase interest in the inner life of the other, for the role we play during a physical encounter – representing our own interests – ceases to apply. This is not only through the absence of physical contact, but above all through meditative reflection, because in order to be able to 'see' beyond the threshold, one must first discard one's selfishness by recognizing it. (This is clearly and pictorially described by the mantras in the first two Class Lessons.)

Whoever cannot readily experience this has other, external means to obtain information about the needs and sensitivities of the other person, and then to motivate oneself in a spiritually-deepened way. One can write a letter, call by telephone or – for many anthroposophists apparently an unforgivable *faux pas* – by digital means for the most necessary things. In my opinion, whoever leads a hygienic inner life has no need to fear occasionally using this latter means of contact, as long as it is done with a sense of proportion and understanding, even if this medium is a gift of the ahrimanic spirits. This is an old subject that has been discussed over and over again in anthroposophical circles, so I'd rather not go into it much here: the question of dealing with so-called social media and with the digital world in general. Rudolf Steiner pointed out that the technical domination of the world will happen in one way or another. It would be naive to think that it can be avoided. It makes more sense to me to be clear about how to use it and to practice this in a timely way. Probably nobody today would think of themselves as Ahriman's servant in the modern world in which karma has placed us if we use a doorbell, enter an elevator, switch on a light or turn on the heating.

I must admit that I am glad to fight Ahriman with his own weapons, in that it provides an easy way for me to contribute to our spiritual work. It's not much different than dealing with the coronavirus. Whether the use of virtual, digital media or the coronavirus will damage our souls depends upon whether in this situation we are at least aware that something else exists besides the purely material, physical-chemical or technical world, and that behind or within all of this something is active that first brought our material world into being and also alters it.

In this situation we might be able to take a new step forward in the social sphere. We could use this physical-social (not spiritual-social!) isolation in order to consider what can be done in the future, when the restrictions are lifted, to develop a new quality of consciousness in our daily contact with each other, which could bring out more of the *essence* of the other and of things. And we could use it to reflect upon how the force of thoughts extends into physical things. As spiritual students, we want to use humanity's fate as an effective therapy.

Starting Point: Consistently Practise Soul Exercises

The often referenced *salutogenesis* – an outwardly gesturing impulse that can offer healing to our fellow human beings – can only take as its starting point for the anthroposophist the consistent practising of the soul exercises, for example as they are described in the book *Knowledge of Higher Worlds and its Attainment*. If until now one has not been able to consistently practise these, the present time offers the best opportunity to do so! For ultimately we are only harming ourselves by not doing so, and by not fighting our complacency and laziness. For it is only in this way that the sources of new epidemics can dry up in the future, and healing powers become effective in one's own organism and in the organism of humanity.

As I have often said – excuse me for repeating myself – the consistent psychical-spiritual work of an individual, or of a few individuals, can have an enormous influence on the spiritual and physical conditions of the world! The emphasis on numbers is not as relevant in the spiritual world as it is on the earth. When someone asks: What can I as one person do to influence world events? – the answer is: everything! If people could only see with physical eyes the effect on the macrocosmic context that the decision and its implementation to consistently practise only one meditation by a single person, then probably no one would hesitate to undertake such an exercise themselves. For the possibilities are enormous! Allow me to give you this as the greatest consolation, as the strongest ray of hope in the present situation. The individual person holds the world's fate in his hands. This is the gift of Christ, who sees the individual I as a deity, who treats it as a deity. We are free beings, and therefore our relationship to the world is in our own hands – in all times and at every moment.

Spiritual life must become a reality in our hearts and thereby in our higher consciousness! We must develop a feeling in our souls for *the true, the beautiful and the good* that resides in this spiritual life.

Suggestions for Spiritual Support for the Ongoing Work in the Branch

> *Admire the beautiful*
> *Care for the true*
> *Venerate the noble*
> *Resolve the good:*
> *It leads humanity*
> *To aims in life*
> *To doing what is right*
> *In feeling at peace*
> *In thinking to light;*
> *And teaches trust*
> *In divine workings*
> *In all that there is*
> *In the universe*
> *In the depths of soul.*

(Rudolf Steiner, *Truth Wrought Words*, GA 40[8])

For this reason I have recommended the above evening prayer as a meditation when beginning branch work, to take place as usual at 6:30 pm on Wednesdays. It was originally given for a child, but its content is appropriate for the oldest among us.

To be conscious of the meaning of these mantric, poetic words – to think the true, thus creating a secure home in your own thinking, to feel the beautiful and develop a chaste admiration and simultaneously a warm love for it, and to resolve and do the good, to make ourselves into steadfast knights for this good in the world – all this leads us to what we need so much, especially in the present situation: *trust in divine workings* in the macrocosmic wide world as well as in the microcosmic inner self. Then we accomplish no less than the kingdom of God, the coming of which we ask for in the Lord's Prayer, be extended to our human surroundings.

This constitutes reality! And if we do this together and at the same time, then we are truly performing – even without physical proximity – a religious ritual.

Now I would like to recommend the following to you: in Rudolf Steiner's Complete Works (GA) volume 267, *Soul Exercises, Volume 1,*[9] there is an exercise concerning development of the sixteen-petal lotus flower that will be familiar to you from *Knowledge of the Higher Worlds and its Attainment.*[10] It is an eight-step exercise, which Rudolf Steiner recommends here (not in *Knowledge of the Higher Worlds*) spread over seven days of the week and – as though made for our branch work – recommends the carrying out of the individual exercises over a period of fourteen days.

I would like to provide the impulse for an experiment that aims at the consistent implementation of psychical exercises. But please feel completely free and take my suggestion as a motivation and not as an obligation! However, the opportunity possibly exists to consistently do these daily exercises if we know that the other friends in our community are also doing them. By the way, in psychical self-training it is certainly permitted to use such mutual motivational methods. Additionally, if we all truly perform this small task over the next weeks, a great force unfolds, not only in our own inner selves, but also for the real presence and action of truth in the outer world.

Although the first exercise is marked for Saturday, I think it is acceptable and sensible to begin with the first exercise on Wednesday evening, the day of the branch meetings, or on the following Thursday morning. Please advise if the need arises to share your experiences or to ask questions.

Another suggestion is that during these fourteen days the first chapter of Rudolf Steiner's book, *The Threshold of the Spiritual World* (GA 17)[11] be reread: 'Concerning the Reliance which may be placed on Thinking; the Nature of the Thinking Soul; and Of Meditation'.

And now a somewhat more unconventional suggestion: that the Foundation Stone verse (GA 260) be spoken, by memory if possible, outside in nature. I don't mean that we should recite it loudly enough for others to hear, but intimately, unheard by others – but not only spoken in thought, letting the words resound in the outer world. (Please take care that you only do this when you cannot be overheard by others. I ask this not to protect you from mockery or derogatory opinions, but rather that in this way there is no danger that others might speak these words in imitation or in vain. For in these exercises it is we who are completely 'naked' and honest in a genuine, natural relationship to our spiritual homeland and the divine beings who prevail in it.)

The experiences that one has when speaking the Foundation Stone verse in nature are incomparably nourishing and sublime. One has the truthful and therefore enormously powerful feeling that cosmic truth is pouring through one's own throat into creation, and in that – in speaking the words – the whole creation speaks them back at the same time. Speaking the truth, this truth of cosmic wisdom is today (one could say, unfortunately) a shattering relief – for oneself, for one's fellow humans, the divine spiritual world and, above all, for the physical world.

One also experiences the true Trinitarian activity in a way that is otherwise not the case in spiritual contemplation. One stands as a human being within this Trinitarian activity – activity that is always present, but for which one becomes to a certain extent co-responsible, co-active, through one's own experience directly on earth. These are only a few inklings of the experiences with which the soul can become permeated. And you can be certain that as long as these exercises can be performed, you will have your own and perhaps other experiences as well.

I have the impression that of all poems, proverbs and mantras the Foundation Stone verse – once experienced in this way – occupies a special position. In any case, in this way we get completely out of our own thoughts and can become directly aware of the reality of the spiritual world flowing through our whole being.

As a mantric conclusion to our branch evening, I would like to recommend the Michael verse 'Victorious Spirit', which shows us the essence of the true spirit of our time and, through its character, not only makes us aware of our contemporary tasks in everyday practical life, but can also give us the necessary will to fulfil them.

> *Victorious spirit*
> *Flame away the impotence*
> *Of timid souls.*
> *Burn up self-interest,*
> *Kindle compassion,*
> *So that selflessness,*
> *As the life-stream of humanity,*
> *Reigns as source*
> *Of spiritual rebirth.*

(From Rudolf Steiner, *Mantric Sayings, Meditations 1903-25*, GA 268.)[12]

I wish you my heartfelt best and am already looking forward to our seeing each other again.

Judith v. Halle

PS: How wonderful that we are united in our community in every situation of life.

III.
THE GREAT DIVERSIONARY MANOEUVRE**

** [Swiss] Publisher's Note to this Appendix: Between the time of Judith von Halle's writing about the coronavirus pandemic in the form of the two letters and the publication of the first edition of this book [in German], which was sold out a few days later, five weeks passed. During that time, developments took place that caused new questions to be asked, to which Judith von Halle refers in this appendix. The original intention was for it to appear in an anthroposophical periodical. However, because none of the magazines to which the piece was offered were disposed to publish it, we decided to make it available here.

Because of this, both the publisher and the readers are faced with the circumstance that the second [German] edition of this book contains a contribution which the first edition lacked. We would be grateful for your understanding. *Joseph Morel, Dornach, 12 May 2020.*

Considered from an objective perspective, a picture emerges from the swirling dust of the corona period. It shows, to those who are able to abandon personal opinions, that the actual force of events has now begun to be unleashed. One could also say: the seeds have borne fruit.

Beyond the actual pandemic or the question about the virus and the illness caused by it, a new theme moves many people, above all in the industrialized and affluent countries, especially in Germany. People seem gradually to have fallen into two basic factions: in one, the initiators and supporters of the measures mandated by the state for the containment of the coronavirus pandemic, and in the other, those who oppose and criticize these measures.

So far, however, only a few seem to be asking themselves questions of the kind that Jonathan Stauffer, for example, is asking. In the Newsletter of the Futurum publishing house, with the title 'Looking back to 1 May 2020', he wonders how in respect to coronavirus he suddenly could have found himself associated ideologically with a community of people 'with whom I have absolutely nothing in common' and that 'the critical questions, the courageous people and the normal and necessary investigations' are only found in 'channels which I have only disputed with from a safe distance'. And he asks, 'What's going on here?'

In any case, it seems obvious that the political establishment and the media, forced into line by the state, allow no room for the 'normal and necessary investigations', nor the corresponding reporting. This indicates that we are dealing with a 'ghost' in respect to coronavirus, 'which manipulates us' – and Stauffer asks what 'our weapons' against this ghost are. He's campaigning for an insight – an embrace of this foreign will – to understand 'what drives our brothers to go "with bombs and guns"' (quoting lyrics by Konstantin Wecker), with which he is referring to the state's methods for containing the pandemic. Although these statements and proposals are appropriate and honourable, they do little to answer his original question.

Jonathan Stauffer rightly observes that 'everything is upside down'. He refers to how so many people within the anthroposophical scene have spoken out during the last days and weeks. Namely, that someone like Wolfgang Wodarg[††] is 'ridiculed and ostracized' whilst Karl Lauterbach[‡‡] – 'who with drums and trumpets wants to make the lockdown even stricter and warns of a second wave, although in Germany and Switzerland there has been no real first wave' – is 'revered'. (Those who have lost a relative, regardless of age, or who do not live in Germany or Switzerland but, for instance, in Spain or Italy, might consider such statements somewhat cynical, hurtful or apathetic.)

[††] Wolfgang Wodarg is a German physician who has criticized the German government's strategy for tackling coronavirus.

[‡‡] Karl Lauterbach is a German scientist and politician of the Social Democratic Party of Germany.

The situation appears to be clear: There, the powerful lobby of panic-mongers, truth twisters and the willing servants of a worldwide health-dictatorship; here, the repressed 'lone fighters who refuse to bow down and who do what is humanly possible', to continue 'their unwavering and intrepid quest' for the 'conclusive truth' – as it says in the Newsletter.

A contrasting image reveals itself from out of the swirling dust: Indeed! We are being manipulated – but not in such an obvious black-and-white way.

The present contribution is in no way intended to give the impression that the questions that many people are asking about the pandemic control measures prescribed by governments worldwide are not justified. It should also not be a plea to accept without objection what the media describes as the difficulty in seeking objective, serious information about coronavirus, or about other political, social or economic questions, or not to look behind the scenes in order to investigate the deeper causes of certain developments! But this article seeks to direct our attention to another aspect, which seems to be little considered, although in my opinion it should be urgently considered.

If we observe the picture more closely, it will be seen that with all the brave protest movements of the present – be they animal rights, protecting the climate or corona protest movements – something terrible is happening below the surface, something subtle and perfidious that takes possession of the good intentions of thousands or even millions of people. The good intentions are not somehow redirected or utilized for other purposes. For the various movements do achieve success in their fields. What is perfidious is that such well-intentioned, justified and necessary initiatives meet with the reaction of the opposition, which is thereby strengthened – which cannot be otherwise and which is basically good. What is really threatening, and somewhat diabolic, is exactly what is intended: i.e., that the wonderful and great enthusiasm that develops within these movements – above all in the younger generation – as well as the complete concentration of the activists, who are so utterly bound up in these movements, ensures that one thing will certainly not occur.

The Awareness of the Central Event of Our Time, the Perception of the Christ Entity as an Etheric Phenomenon

But the future of the individual and our humanity depends on this perception! For through it everything that is urgently needed now will become possible: Only through it can human beings arrange their deeds on earth so they don't stand on feet of clay. For Christ touches and stirs the individual soul in such a way that a person experiences a complete transformational impulse in his whole being. Such a person gains a new vision of the human being, of his genesis and purpose, of the total sense of his incarnation and of the world, and not least the needs of humanity's habitat, the earth. The individual also no longer needs to pretend and, through all kinds of tricks, motivate himself to act according to Christian-anthroposophical concepts, embracing what others may want, for example. Such conduct necessarily flees from his or her soul. Through the encounter with Christ and the resulting insights, an individual can become a reliable member of a new, sustainable and enduring community. Furthermore, through the direct inner contact with that spirit who once called himself *the truth* and *the life*, the individual is able to develop true concepts of the things and processes beyond and on this side of the threshold. The encounter with the Being of Christ elevates the individual's thought life to otherwise hardly-attainable heights of understanding and thus to a healthy capacity for humility toward the godly, love toward the divine and love and peace toward his or her fellow human beings. And last but not least: the 'knowledge of evil' and its intentions (according to Rudolf Steiner the task of the present fifth post-Atlantian cultural epoch) can only be attained if one experiences something of that entity – in a truly self-experiential way – against which that evil is directed. Only through the all-decisive encounter with Christ is one freed from one's narrow angle of vision, which previously distorted one's view of greater contexts, especially when you thought you were seeing the greater contexts clearly, but then finally were left in oppressive perplexity.

For evil's web is so wide, spread over every area of earthly existence, that the person who begins to investigate its roots inevitably gets stuck in the undergrowth of innumerable details and entanglements, and at some point feels spun into a cocoon from which neither he nor the rest of humanity can escape – that is, if 'the light of the world' (John: 8,12) does not show him the way out of the web.

However, for the perception of a being that does not reveal itself physically and in sensual work but etherically, certain conditions are necessary. The spiritual eyes of those who are imprisoned in a wholly sensory existence, who concentrate solely on the exterior events in the world, remain closed.

And this is just what is now happening: 'Yes, those brotherhoods ... who wish to banish the human soul to the materialistic sphere ... are striving to let the Christ pass by unnoticed in the twentieth century, not to let his coming as an ethereal individuality become noticeable by human beings.' Instead, they wish to install 'a different individuality, who did not even appear in the flesh, but only as an etheric individuality, but of a strong ahrimanic nature'.§§ Sorat is meant – the sun-demon, whose third uprising we have been experiencing since the end of the twentieth century. We are living within its effects.

This entity is not witless. It doesn't always act where expected. Mostly, it acts where *not* expected.

---

§§ Rudolf Steiner: GA 178, lecture of 18 November 1917. Published in English as *Secret Brotherhoods and the Mystery of the Human Double*, Rudolf Steiner Press 2011.

Thus, Goethe has his Mephistopheles confess to Faust as follows:

MEPHISTOPHELES (*Seriously*)

When the Lord God – and I know why as well –
Banished us from the air to deepest deeps,
There, where round and round the glow of Hell,
An eternal inward self-fuelled fire leaps,
We found we were too brightly illuminated,
Quite crowded, and uncomfortably situated.
All the devils fell to fits of coughing,
The vents above them and beneath them puffing,
Hell swollen with the sulphur's stench and acid,
Gave out its gas! The bubble was so massive,
That soon the level surface of the earth,
Thick as it was, was forced to crack and burst.
So we all gained another mountain from it,
And what was ground, before, now is summit.
From this they deduced the truest law,
Turn lowest into highest, to be sure,
Since we escaped from fiery prison there,
To excessive power in the freer air:
An open mystery, yet well concealed,
And only late to the people revealed.   (Part II, 4)

Indeed: 'Everything is upside down'!

The insidious plan, the well-kept secret, is that thoroughly-Christian values, ideals, motives, conscious actions and energy be misused for purely physical aspects of sensory life.

And – what must be admitted for better or worse – the movements against climate change or the current protest movements against the restrictions of certain aspects of life during the coronavirus period, are ultimately sensory-related movements. These are without doubt important ecological, political, economic and social questions. *But never about spiritual questions.* Nobody protests, either openly on the streets or digitally on the internet, that the decisive event for the individual and for all of humanity is not mentioned with one single syllable – is not in the least bit noticed!

The inestimable loss of *freedom in spiritual/cultural life* is not even mentioned. For that spiritual life which is based on a true knowledge of the Christ entity is not even missed at all. The criticism is mostly directed at the loss of 'civil rights'. In the sphere of individual rights – if one follows the concept of social threefolding – one should speak of *equality*, just as in economic affairs it about *fraternity*.

Don't let the swirling dust get in your eyes! Not only the ordinary politician or the classic virologist, but even a Wolfgang Wodarg does not consider the spiritual world in his research, reports and judgments. All physical events and manifestations, however, derive from this spiritual world. The appearance of viruses is not seen – whether in the public or in citizens' initiatives, regardless of orientation – in connection with processes that take place in the spiritual realm.

That we live with viruses is an attitude of mind that nobody, especially not the anthroposophical spiritual student, should agree or be satisfied with. For as such, the spiritual student possesses the insight that there are many different revelations from many different spiritual beings within the sensory world, which in their moral quality and aims are completely contrary, and for this reason should be recognized and differentiated. On this basis an anthroposophist can easily recognize that nothing pathological (such as the coronavirus) can ensue from a *good* divine spirituality. Rather, the existence of life-threatening or 'only' illness-causing pathogens is a sign that in the present widespread pandemic, the shifting and workings of a sub-sensory spiritual power is misunderstood and therefore not banished. The discussion about tightening or easing social restrictions is therefore – as justified as it is – missing the point as long as this essential aspect is not taken into account.

In that kingdom whose coming we ask in the *Lord's Prayer* – the world from which our immortal true being derives – there are no bacteria and viruses! Human pathological bacteria and viruses are products of sick, antagonistic spirituality. They release poisons; physical, psychical and spiritual poisons. To want to live with them in lasting coexistence and to accept them as natural components of human existence and development would mean that human beings have agreed to the stagnation of their spirit, that they have given up their will to differentiate good from evil, health from sickness, morality from immorality – and, on the basis of such knowledge, to develop into a being fit for the future.

That these physical manifestations of immoral spirituality (such as viruses) are present in our world is a fact. That the human being must live and deal with them as long as people are not able to prevent their threats by a highly developed spiritual lifestyle, is also a fact. But our method for dealing with them is only successful if we learn to recognize the essence of the various sensory manifestations and are able to react appropriately. For this, the ability to differentiate is necessary – however, this ability is not possible without progress in the field of spiritual knowledge.

Certainly, human beings can use all that intends to hinder them to their 'altruistic advantage' by transforming these aspects within themselves (by knowledge of the beings that seek to hinder them) so that these beings can no longer hinder the individual. Nevertheless, certain other spiritual impulses which intend to hinder the human being's higher development *remain*, and among them is coronavirus. So, individuals should ask themselves: Where can I obtain the capacity to recognize the essence of the sensory manifestations that I *need to* recognize in order to *be able* to transform them within myself – insofar as a transformation is necessary?

If we look again at the protest movements with which many anthroposophists sympathize or also participate in, it becomes clear that there is something else involved which has not yet become apparent, at least not as distinctly or to the same intensity, as in the animal rights or climate change movements. Within the movements against the state-imposed coronavirus measures, there are quite a number of people whose behaviour and view of humanity run counter to the basic principles of an anthroposophist, as Jonathan Stauffer has also noted. At the same time there are large numbers of people in these movements who represent neither anthroposophical nor extremist views. Thus this protest movement consists of a potpourri of fears, assertions, objections and complaints.

The call for self-determination, for *freedom*, is what unites all the different people in these protest movements.

But what kind of freedom is meant? Or rather, what is our concept of freedom?

With due respect to the individual, in view of the growing number of people joining these protest movements, it is necessary to speak of the basic under-lying reason that is the real cause of many people's discontent. In the age of consciousness soul devel-opment, human beings have deeply rooted psychi-cal-spiritual needs which result from their basic state of mind and therefore differ from the needs of previ-ous ages that were determined by the sentient soul or the intellectual soul ages. At present the human being has not yet been able to subdue these needs. They are still there, and will become more urgent so long as we are unable to subdue them.

Human needs in the consciousness soul age con-sist in a desire for the activity of one's own con-sciousness soul, that is, for a cognitive encounter with reality – with that which both gives us a genuine insight into the connections of the world as a whole and instills real life. In this age, one could say, in response to the ahrimanic spirits' attack on the individual personality since the year 1879, the Christ is at our side – internally perceptible today – to help satisfy the aforementioned needs. Although everyone feels these needs distinctly, many people are not conscious of them, so they become increasingly anxious. The individual is thirsty for something which they don't recognize. This leads to confusion and restlessness, to a general malaise.

Due to the fact that the spiritual reason for this malaise and dissatisfaction is unknown – because the spiritual domain is widely considered to be nonexistent or a matter of personal belief – we seek for the reason in every other field except the correct one. Thus, in one protest movement the most varied reasons for protest may be found. Therefore the protest, like the painfully felt but unnameable subconscious deficits, has a general character and is directed against the general public or its representatives or their presumed influencers.

It cannot be dismissed out of hand – and Rudolf Steiner's quote above confirms this – that since the last third of the nineteenth century there have been serious attempts by certain interest groups to drive humanity into unfavorable waters. But even if within these protest movements things are repeated that come from people in the know, there is still a dangerous potential here. For if the means do not exist in individuals to examine such claims from within their own spiritual insight or to understand them, they are of little use. But they can be harmful, because in this way fear arises – fear of an unknown enemy, an invisible threat. Thereby the protest movements do exactly what they accuse others of doing (surely not unjustly), by using excessive methods and one-sided information to incite fear.

No government in the world, regardless of how criminal it may be, can be blamed that the means for knowledge in the individual soul are not sufficient to clearly understand such circumstances; because no one except the individual human being is to blame for this. (At most one could argue that, because so many human 'I's have not sought the spirit during the past 150 years, in the meantime humanity as such has created conditions that make a spiritual understanding of events very difficult for the individual in these times. But that is a more spiritual viewpoint, related namely to humanity's karma, and because the majority of the protesters probably have little knowledge of the reality and the spiritual mechanisms of karma, their protest refers as little to this overall human karmic responsibility for present world events as to their own individual responsibility in this regard.)

So looking for scapegoats begins. And if some are found among them who really serve the plot of the sub-sensory spiritual forces against the strengthening of humanity – it is like the proverbial blind chicken who looks around so much that it finally finds a seed – the knowledge of *why* is still lacking; the right words are lacking, because one is oneself sleeping in respect to the spirit, so no other outlet is found other than joining a wave of protests. But the exterior protest is totally ineffective against such forces and their manifestations, for real effectiveness can only be brought about by comprehension. First of all, there must be the acquisition of the appropriate means of knowledge, and secondly, based on this, the higher ratio and the resulting decisions on further action.

Those who protest in mass protest movements against the villains but deny the living spirit, put the means of manipulation into the hands of those villains themselves. You make yourself the cue ball in a game whose rules you don't understand because you don't read the game's instructions – because you refuse to learn to read.

Thus the criticism seldom hits its target, but remains diffuse and ultimately leads to the demand for personal freedom, the deprivation of which one feels painfully – and thereby hits the bullseye. However, what one feels as deprivation of personal freedom is in reality the yoke of the self-responsible unfreedom of one's own higher spirituality, which is subject to the denial of itself, namely the spirit – and thus also of Christ.

Sometimes the impression arises that even among anthroposophists the reality of this higher spirituality is not taken to be completely real. For those who remind us of it are quickly classified as 'gnostics', which probably means that they are somewhat unworldly, not having their feet completely on the ground regarding current reality – and by now this probably also includes Rudolf Steiner.

Everything is Upside Down

In these upside down times one should nevertheless recall words from Rudolf Steiner – indeed precisely for this reason – which again remind us of that being of which we are so reluctant to be reminded today, because it makes us feel circumscribed in our self-image as an enlightened and completely self-sufficient free spirit:

> We should not be able to grasp the thought of freedom without the thought of Redemption through Christ: only then is the thought of freedom justified. If we want to be free, we must bring the offering of thanks to Christ for our freedom! Only then can we really perceive it. And those who consider it beneath their dignity to thank Christ for it, should realize that human opinions have no significance in face of cosmic facts, and that one day they will very willingly acknowledge that their freedom was won by Christ. (GA 131, lecture of 14 October 1911.)[13]

If we internalize the truth to the point of feeling that, in the freedom of our individuality – in the freedom of the spiritual entity which we in truth are – nobody can curtail and control this by external circumstances – also not through the fact that we are forced by state decrees to limit our contacts or going out – then we are much better able to discuss the sense or senselessness of such government-imposed restrictions on a solid foundation and with inner calmness. If not, the protest quickly descends to a path it should have avoided. Petty personal egotism mixes with justified arguments. Debates about politically decreed measures become central, whilst the actual (spiritual) causes of the viral pandemic, the role of the spirit of the present time, the knowledge of Christ and his adversary is completely pushed aside.

The discussion becomes heated, the resistance reflexive. Let us observe ourselves! Even in anthroposophical contributions the diction often imitates scenes of war. We discuss the right 'weapons' in 'battle' against the 'corona lie'. The 'undaunted lone warriors', who will 'never concede' over a 'power grab': the question of 'who will be victorious', and much more.

But when furore, revulsion and hate circulate in the soul, when we consider such emotions justified and admit them – whether in deeds, feelings or thoughts – because we believe we are experiencing injustice and are therefore in the right, then that being who sacrificed himself for us on the cross in order to bring love to the world is not in accordance with us. What unites us in inciting fear and crude conspiracy theories and using scientists' contradictions is undeniably the absence of Christ in our consciousness – the forgetting to use the indispensable means of spiritual(!)-science.

The spirits which we have to do with today are 'To the excess of the dominion of free air' (Faust), and remain mostly unknown. Our thoughts, which they try to influence to the extent that we believe the enemy to be clearly localized and identified, float in this sphere of free air. This conviction is their most delicious prey. They misuse our intentions.

They incorporate themselves not only in 'our fear or our complacency' (J. Stauffer), in moral cowardice before an – democratically elected or not – authority, but if the central spiritual events and entities are ignored, they also incorporate themselves in our fiery efforts against them!

Humanity, which is falling into two camps of opinion is – seen from within – not really divided. It is united in falling for the great diversionary manoeuvre. The coronavirus itself is not the great diversionary manoeuvre, rather everything that follows. The attention and forces of millions of people – as different in opinions and intentions as they may be – are equally bound to let the central event of our time, which could make us the legitimate representatives of our time, *pass by unnoticed.*

If we who by grace of destiny know anthroposophy allow ourselves to be blown away by a storm of indignation – composed of strong gusts of wind that come from various directions and lose ourselves in liberation skirmishes – or if we don't even try to read the *signs of the times* (GA 346, lecture of 12 September 1924[14]), but in a childish, naive way believe in 'preparing now for the future' by 'entertaining the idea of celebrating the re-opening, perhaps start planning for it' (*Anthroposophy Worldwide*, 5/2020), and in this way completely ignore the work of gaining knowledge, then the spiritual world will have to seek its helpers among those who are unaware of spiritual-scientific concepts, but who nonetheless strive for a real connection to the spiritual world; namely among those who, for example, tirelessly pray, or such who do not fear being laughed at when bearing witness to their near-death experiences or about their personal encounters with the reality of God. But then we will also be responsible for the fact that in the near future wholly different, much worse plagues than a SARS-CoV-2 pandemic will afflict us. Thus, a different way must be found to deal with the current challenges.

Humanity is forgetting the God within. (See Rudolf Steiner: 'For the Berliner Friends', in GA 268[15]). The anthroposophist should be conscious of this. When he 'fights', he should fight for this God within by beginning to direct his or her own view, and possibly that of his fellow human beings, to this God within.

> That is anthroposophy's great responsibility. Anthroposophy has sprung from a knowledge of the necessity for an advanced preparation for something which will come, but which could be overlooked and suppressed. Anthroposophy has the task of bringing about an understanding of the spiritual forces developing in man. If these forces are suppressed humanity will sink deeper into materialism. […]
>
> Not for nothing has man been placed in the physical world; for it is where we must acquire what leads us to an understanding of the Christ-Impulse! For all the souls now living, anthroposophy is the preparation for the Christ-Event [in the etheric world]. This preparation is necessary. [...] It will therefore be an important omission if people who have the opportunity of elevating themselves during this century to the Christ-Event do not wish to do so.

Only if we consider anthroposophy in this way and inscribe it in our souls, can we feel what it is for each human soul and what it should be for all humanity.' (GA 116, Lecture of 8 February 1910.[16])

Judith von Halle
Berlin, 11 May 2020

Appendix

The Eight Soul Exercises by Rudolf Steiner

For the Days of the Week
The person must pay careful attention to certain psychical activities which ordinarily are carried on carelessly and inattentively. There are eight such activities.

It is naturally best to undertake only one exercise at a time, for a week or two, for example, then the second, and so on, then beginning over. Meanwhile it is best, however, for the eighth exercise to be done every day. One then gradually achieves self-knowledge and also sees what progress has been made. Later, beginning with Saturday, one exercise lasting for about five minutes may be added daily to the eighth, so that the relevant exercise will fall on the same day. Thus on Saturdays, the Thoughts exercise; Sundays, the Resolves; Mondays, Talking; Tuesdays, Actions; Wednesdays, the Deeds; and so on.

Saturday
Paying attention to one's mental images (thoughts).
Think only significant thoughts. Learn little by little to separate in one's thoughts the essential from the nonessential, the eternal from the transitory, truth from mere opinion. When listening to others, try to be quite still inwardly, foregoing all assent, and still

more all unfavourable judgments (criticism, rejection), even in one's thoughts and feelings.
This is so-called: *'Right Thinking'*.

Sunday
To decide on even the most insignificant matter only after fully reasoned deliberation. All unthinking behaviour, all meaningless actions, should be kept distant from the soul. One should always have well-determined reasons for everything. And one should definitely abstain from doing anything for which there is no significant reason. Once one is convinced of the rightness of a decision, one must hold fast to it, with inner steadfastness.

This may be called: *'Right Judgment'* – having been formed independently of sympathies and antipathies.

Monday
Talking. Only what has sense and meaning should come from the lips of one striving for higher development. Talking for the sake of talking, to kill time, for example, is in this sense harmful.

The usual kind of conversation, a disjointed medley of remarks, should be avoided. This does not mean shutting oneself off from intercourse with others; it is precisely in such a situation that talk should gradually become meaningful. Have a thoughtful attitude to every question and answer, taking all aspects into account. Never speak without a reason. Prefer silence. Try not to talk too much or too little. First listen quietly, then reflect on what has been said.

This exercise is called: *'Right words'*.

Tuesday
External actions. These should not be disturbing for other people. When an occasion calls for action out of one's inner self (conscience), consider carefully how you can best do so for the good of the whole, for the lasting happiness of all others, for the eternal.

When you do things on your own, on your own initiative, consider thoroughly beforehand the effect of your actions.

This is called: *'The Right Deed'*.

Wednesday
The organization of life. Live naturally and spiritually. Don't be absorbed by the external trivialities of life. Avoid everything that causes turmoil and haste in life. Don't be hasty, but don't be indolent either. Consider life as a means for working towards higher development and behave accordingly.

This is called: *'Right Standpoint'*.

Thursday
Human striving. Take care to do nothing that lies beyond your powers, but also leave nothing undone which lies within them.

Look beyond the everyday, the momentary, and set yourself goals (ideals) related to the highest duties of a human being, for example to develop, in the sense of these prescribed exercises, so that afterwards you are more able to help and advise others, though perhaps not in the immediate future.

This can be summed up as: *'Let all the foregoing exercises become habitual'*.

Friday

Strive to learn as much as possible from life. Nothing happens without it giving us occasion to gain experiences that are useful for life. If you do something wrongly or imperfectly, it becomes an opportunity for doing something that is similarly right or perfect later.

If you see others acting, observe them with a view to a similar goal (but not unkindly). And you do nothing without looking back on experiences that can help you in your decisions and actions.

One can learn from everyone, even from children if one is attentive.

This exercise is called: *'Right Memory'* (that is, remembering what has been learned from previous experiences).

Summary

Turn your gaze inward from time to time, if only for five minutes daily at the same time. In so doing you should submerge within yourself, carefully consult with yourself, examine and formulate your life's principles, think through your knowledge — or its lack — consider your duties, think about the content and true purpose of life, feel genuinely displeased by your mistakes and imperfections. In a word: seek what is essential and enduring, and seriously set yourself corresponding goals, for example virtues to be acquired. (Do not fall into the error of thinking that you have done something well, but keep on striving, following the highest examples.)

This exercise is called: *'Right Contemplation'*

Notes

1. 'Corona Pandemic – Aspects and Perspectives' by Matthias Girke and Georg Soldner, Medical Section, School of Spiritual Science, Dornach, 19 March 2020. An English version can be found in the book *Perspectives and Initiatives in the Times of Coronavirus*, Edited by Ueli Hurter and Justus Wittich, Rudolf Steiner Press 2020.

2. See Rudolf Steiner, lecture of 5 May 1914 in *The Presence of the Dead on the Spiritual Path*, Anthroposophic Press 1990.

3. For these quotations see Rudolf Steiner, *On Epidemics*, Rudolf Steiner Press 2011.

4. See Rudolf Steiner, *The Fall of the Spirits of Darkness* (GA 177), Rudolf Steiner Press 1993.

5. Rudolf Steiner, *From Jesus to Christ* (GA 131), Rudolf Steiner Press 1973.

6. Judith von Halle, *Illness and Healing*, Temple Lodge Publishing 2008.

7. For indications of the spiritual background of that war see my book *Die Sieben Mysteriendramen Rudolf Steiners*, Dornach 2016, p. 95ff.

8. Rudolf Steiner, *Wahrspruchworte* (GA 40), 9th edition, Dornach 2005, p. 324. English edition: *Truth-Wrought Words*, Anthroposophic Press 1979.

9. Rudolf Steiner, *Soul Exercises, 1904-1924* (GA 26), 'For the Days of the Week', p. 11. SteinerBooks 2014.

10. Rudolf Steiner, *Knowledge of the Higher Worlds, How is it Achieved?* (GA 10), Rudolf Steiner Press 2004. See Appendix.

11. Rudolf Steiner, *The Threshold of the Spiritual World* (GA 17), Anthroposophical Publishing Co. 1956. Available in: *A Way of Self Knowledge And The Threshold Of The Spiritual World*, SteinerBooks 2006.

12. Rudolf Steiner, *Mantrische Sprüche. Seelenübungen Band II* (GA 268), Dornach 1999, p. 73 ('Sieghafter Geist...', Meditationsworte, die den Willen ergreifen). English edition: *Mantric*

Sayings, Meditations 1903 – 1925, Soul exercises, 1903-1925, SteinerBooks 2015.

[13] Rudolf Steiner, *From Jesus to Christ,* Rudolf Steiner Press 1973. Lecture of 14 October 1911.

[14] See *The Book of Revelation and the Work of the Priest,* Rudolf Steiner Press 1998.

[15] See Rudolf Steiner, *Mantric Sayings, Meditations 1903-1925,* SteinerBooks 2015.

[16] See *The Christ Impulse and the Development of Ego-Consciousness,* Rudolf Steiner Press 2014.

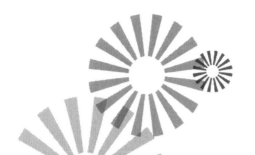

A note from the publisher

For more than a quarter of a century, **Temple Lodge Publishing** has made available new thought, ideas and research in the field of spiritual science.

Anthroposophy, as founded by Rudolf Steiner (1861-1925), is commonly known today through its practical applications, principally in education (Steiner-Waldorf schools) and agriculture (biodynamic food and wine). But behind this outer activity stands the core discipline of spiritual science, which continues to be developed and updated. True science can never be static and anthroposophy is living knowledge.

Our list features some of the best contemporary spiritual-scientific work available today, as well as introductory titles. So, visit us online at **www.templelodge.com** and join our emailing list for news on new titles.

If you feel like supporting our work, you can do so by buying our books or making a direct donation (we are a non-profit/ charitable organisation).

office@templelodge.com

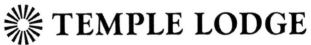

TEMPLE LODGE

For the finest books of Science and Spirit